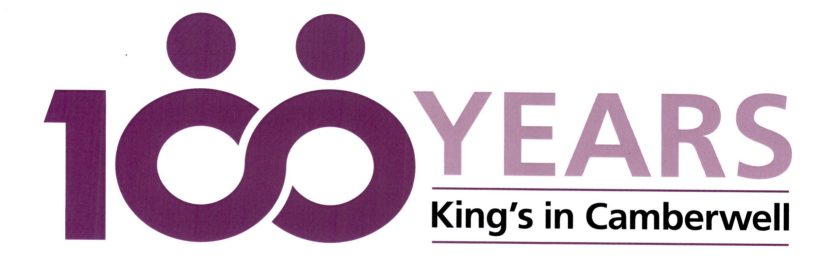

KING'S COLLEGE HOSPITAL CELEBRATING 100 YEARS

A Centenary Souvenir Publication

By Emma Pomfret

Published by King's College Hospital,
Denmark Hill, London, SE5 9RS

© King's College Hospital

2013

Archive images courtesy of King's College London Archives

Page 29 photographs (Q 27814) (Q 27819) © Imperial War Museums
All other photos and images are property of King's College Hospital

Written by Emma Pomfret
Designed by Nicola Gregory

Printed in the UK by Firstpoint Print Victoria
160-162 Vauxhall Bridge Road
London SW1V 2RA.

First Edition
ISBN: 978-0-9926043-1-8

10 9 8 7 6 5 4 3 2 1

A catalogue record for this book is available from the British Library

Typeset
Frutiger LT Std

Contents

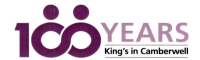

KING'S COLLEGE HOSPITAL FAST FACTS OF TODAY

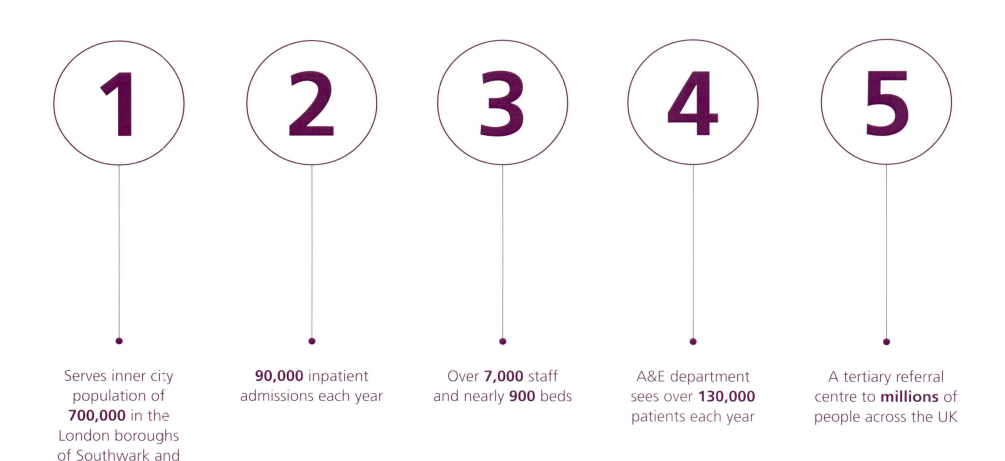

1 Serves inner city population of **700,000** in the London boroughs of Southwark and Lambeth

2 **90,000** inpatient admissions each year

3 Over **7,000** staff and nearly **900** beds

4 A&E department sees over **130,000** patients each year

5 A tertiary referral centre to **millions** of people across the UK

KING'S COLLEGE HOSPITAL FAST FACTS OF TODAY

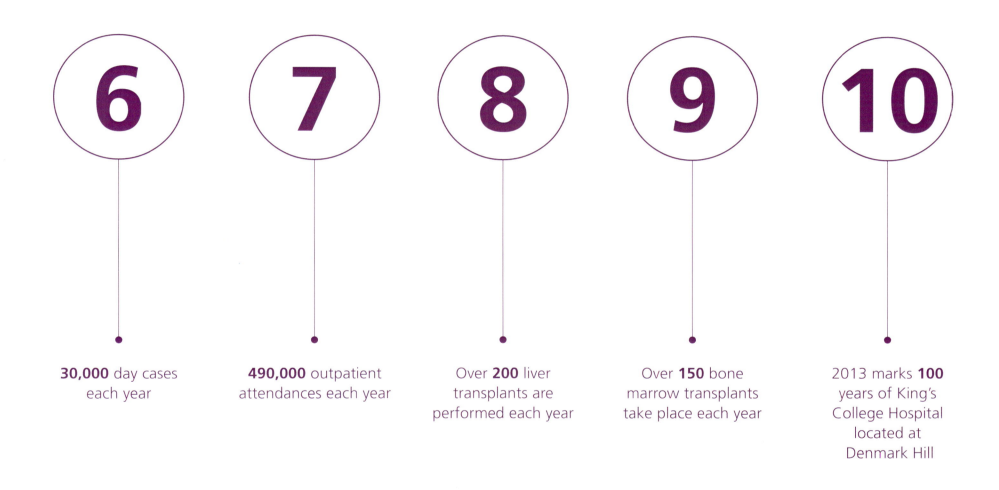

6 — **30,000** day cases each year

7 — **490,000** outpatient attendances each year

8 — Over **200** liver transplants are performed each year

9 — Over **150** bone marrow transplants take place each year

10 — 2013 marks **100** years of King's College Hospital located at Denmark Hill

Chapter 1

THE FOUNDATIONS OF KING'S COLLEGE HOSPITAL

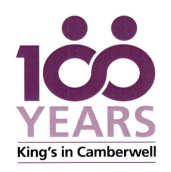

THE FOUNDATIONS OF
KING'S COLLEGE HOSPITAL

Founded as a teaching hospital in 1840, King's College Hospital has placed the local community at its heart ever since it opened its doors in a former workhouse on Portugal Street near Lincoln's Inn Fields in Holborn, and since its **move to Camberwell 100 years ago**. As the community's needs have changed, King's has changed with them

———

In 1840, when the first King's College Hospital opened on Portugal Street, Holborn was nothing like it is today. There was no hustle and bustle of business but dimly lit, squalid, crime-ridden streets and over-crowded slums rife with disease, including cholera. Within two years, King's was treating 1290 inpatients with just 120 beds; the hospital management had to ask medics *"to use all their efforts to prevent the necessity of having two or more patients in one bed."*

In *A History of Britain's Hospitals*, Dr G Barry and Lesley A Carruthers describe King's on Portugal Street as *"located in one of the worst slum districts in London... patients multiplied tenfold to over 30,000 within ten years making relocation essential, accentuated by the pressure of 'noxious gases' issuing from the corpses rotting in the adjacent burial ground."*

A second purpose-built hospital opened on the same site in 1861 with almost twice the number of beds. But by the 1880s a social shift was underway; modernisation was rolling through the Strand and Holborn area. The slums around the hospital were being cleared and replaced by grand new streets

– Holborn Viaduct among them – and businesses. The Strand area lost a third of its residents in 20 years. So King's was seeing fewer patients from central London and more patients from south London – Camberwell, Brixton, Peckham, Dulwich and Nunhead. By 1892 a House of Lords Select Committee advised that a large general hospital be built in Camberwell.

In 1903 it was confirmed that King's would be moving four miles from Holborn to Denmark Hill in Camberwell, its present site. The land – 12 acres – was donated by Lord Hambleden of the W H Smith family. King Edward VII laid the foundation stone for the new building on July 20, 1909. As the hospital was built, the *Daily Chronicle* newspaper described the scene to its readers: *"It is a palace of light and knowledge for those who will find in it healing for their sickness and comfort for their pain… a welcome sight to the eyes of hundreds of thousands of South Londoners."*

But before opening in mid-1913, King's still needed to raise around £125,000 (around £12m equivalent in 2013). A fundraising pamphlet appealed to wealthy donors to name a bed for £1,000 or a ward for £10,000.

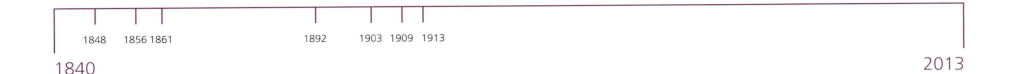

1848   1856 1861   1892   1903 1909 1913

1840   2013

The appeal graciously recognised the more cash-strapped residents of Camberwell: *"It must not be forgotten that the inhabitants of the district immediately adjacent to the new site are very poor and such monetary help as they are able to give to the project can be but small."*

On July 26, 1913 King George V opened the new hospital with Queen Mary. Designed by William Pite, the hospital had 300 beds, four operating theatres and open-plan wards designed for maximum ventilation. Press reports marvelled at the glittering modernity: miles of wiring and piping, the hospital's own diesel-powered electricity and only the second internal phone system in the UK.

From its foundation, King's has been a teaching hospital. Generations of medical and dental students have passed through King's wards and medical school. King's also founded the first nursing school in the country. In 1840 the hospital had one matron and just three untrained nurses. But in 1848 Robert Bentley Todd, the first Dean of King's, founded the first Church of England Nursing Sisterhood, the Sisterhood of Saint John the Evangelist – better known as St John's House. In 1856, nurses from St John's House set up the first nursing school at King's, three years before Florence Nightingale established her training school at St Thomas' Hospital.

KING'S COLLEGE HOSPITAL, PORTUGAL STREET
The second King's – purpose-built at Lincoln's Inn Fields in Holborn

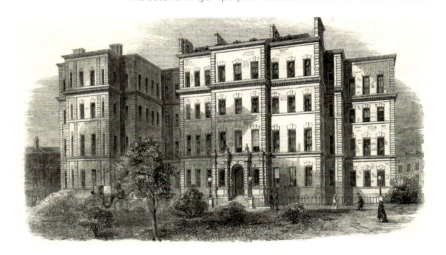

Robert Bentley Todd was instrumental in founding King's College Hospital. He revolutionised teaching at the Medical School and nursing in the hospital and made King's one of the best 19th century hospitals in London.

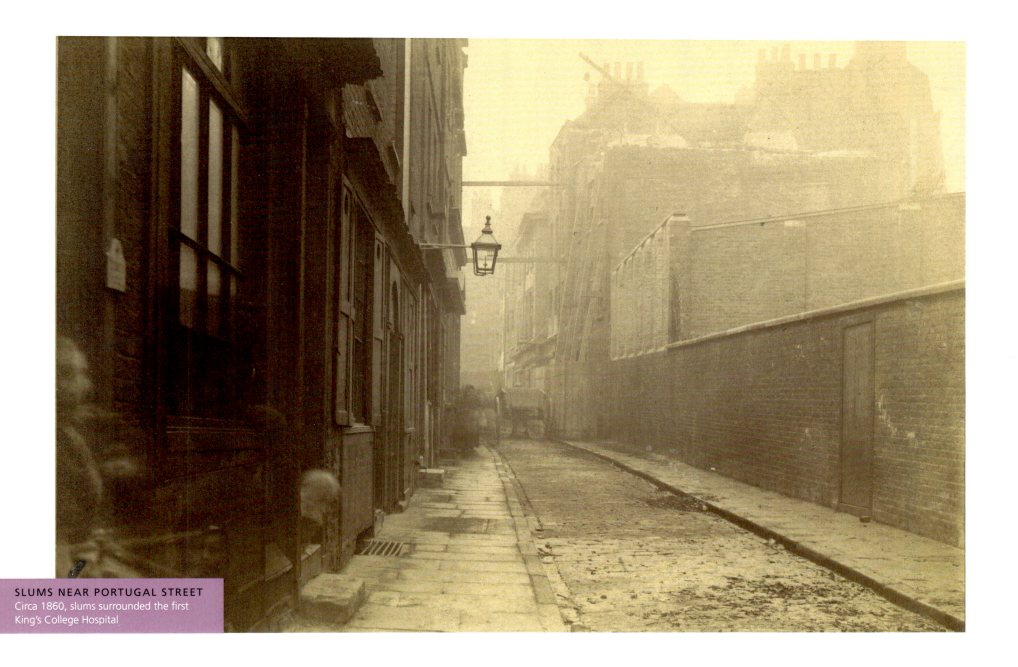

SLUMS NEAR PORTUGAL STREET
Circa 1860, slums surrounded the first
King's College Hospital

THE SITES: OLD AND NEW.

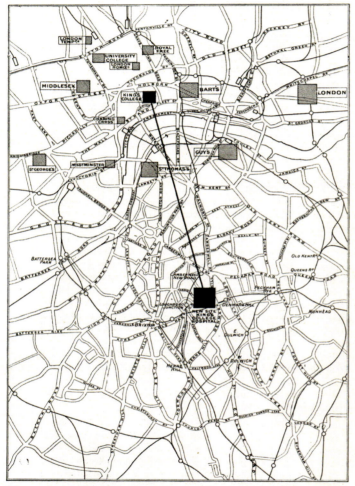

The above map of the West Central and Southern Districts of London indicates the position of King's College Hospital to-day and of the new Hospital. The former building, in Lincoln's Inn Fields, occupies what is practically a "depopulated" area. The new King's College Hospital at Denmark Hill is being built in the heart of a district where a million and a half of very poor people are unprovided with hospital accommodation.

MAP OF THE OLD AND NEW SITE
A fund-raising booklet, circa 1913, explained why King's was moving from central to south London and appealed for donations to the removal fund

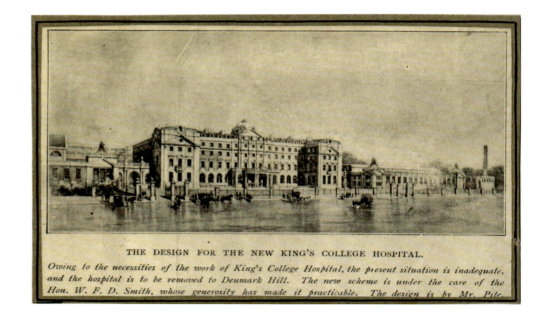

THE DESIGN FOR THE NEW KING'S COLLEGE HOSPITAL.
Owing to the necessities of the work of King's College Hospital, the present situation is inadequate, and the hospital is to be removed to Denmark Hill. The new scheme is under the care of the Hon. W. F. D. Smith, whose generosity has made it practicable. The design is by Mr. Pite.

THE DESIGN FOR THE NEW KING'S COLLEGE HOSPITAL
This sketch, circa 1905, shows William Pite's design for the new hospital

APPEALING FOR FUNDS

This 1915 fundraising pamphlet featured famous surgeon Joseph Lister and suggested levels of donations to suit every budget

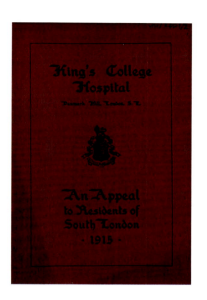

FUNDRAISING COOKERY BOOK

1911 - The Friends of King's published several recipe books sold in aid of the hospital and featuring recipes donated by the Ladies Association. *"The compilers desire to convey their thanks to all those ladies who have so kindly furnished material for the production of this work"*

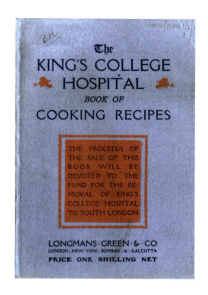

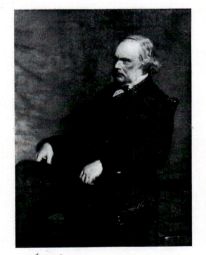

Joseph Lister

THE LATE LORD LISTER,
who was for thirty-five years associated with King's College Hospital, and elaborated there his epoch-making discovery of the Antiseptic principles applied to Surgery.

How you can help the Hospital

If you cannot give

A BLOCK (£20,000); *or*

A WARD (£10,000);

or endow

A BED (£1,000); *or*

A COT (£500);

will you become

A LIFE GOVERNOR, by a donation of not less than £31 10s.; *or*

A GOVERNOR, by an annual subscription of not less than £3 3s.; *or*

AN ANNUAL SUBSCRIBER or DONOR of any smaller sum?

Subscriptions, donations, etc., will be gladly received and acknowledged by the SECRETARY, KING'S COLLEGE HOSPITAL, DENMARK HILL, LONDON, S.E.

9

IN AID OF THE FUND FOR THE REMOVAL OF

Spiced Beef.

¼ lb. Salt.
½ oz. Saltpetre.
¼ oz. Allspice.
½ oz. black Pepper.
¼ lb. brown Sugar.

Thoroughly mix and boil these ingredients in 2 qts. of water and pour hot upon a piece of beef in a glazed jar : let it remain for a fortnight. It must be kept under the pickle with a weight. *N.B.*—The flank cut from the end of the sirloin is very suitable. After being boiled it should be pressed flat and glazed when cold. The pickle may be boiled up and used again.

F. AUSTIN.

To Cure Hams (1).

1 lb. coarse Sugar.
1 lb. Salt.
1 oz. Bay Salt.
1 oz. black Pepper.
1 oz. Saltpetre.
1 oz. Juniper Berries (well bruised).

Mix all together and lay on the hams. When it dissolves baste daily for a month.

MRS. JOHN SAVAGE.

To Cure Hams (2).

2 Hams (20 lbs. each) and 2 Shoulders.

Rub in salt and pepper for 3 days ; then put in pickle. If very cold weather, hang 3 days before salting.

For the Pickle.

4 lbs. brown Sugar.
2 ozs. Sal Prunella.
4 lbs. Treacle.
2 ozs. Bay Salt.
4 lbs. common Salt.
1 cup of Vinegar.

64

KING'S COLLEGE HOSPITAL TO SOUTH LONDON.

Let them lie 1 month, during which the pickle must be thrown over them with a spoon once a day. After the end of the month take them out of the pickle and put into cold water for 24 hours, then hang up to dry.

MRS. DOUGLAS SMITH.

To Cure Hams (3).

1 lb. Bay Salt.
½ lb. common Salt.
2 ozs. Saltpetre.
1 oz. black Pepper (powdered).

Beat all these very fine, then rub the ham (about 20 lbs.) very well and let it lie 4 days, turning it every day, then pour upon it 1 lb. of treacle. Wash it every day with the liquor, and let it stand a month; then steep it in cold water 24 hours, and hang up to dry.

N.B.—This pickle will afterwards cure tongues for drying or immediate use.

MRS. PLAYFAIR.

To Cure Tongues.

1 oz. Saltpetre.
½ oz. black Pepper.
3 ozs. coarse Sugar.
2 ozs. Juniper Berries.
6 ozs. Salt.

Rub the above ingredients well into the tongue (about 7 lbs.) and let it remain in the pickle for a fortnight. Then drain it, tie it up in brown paper, and have it smoked for about 20 days over a wood fire—or it may be boiled out of the pickle.

MRS. VACHELL.

65

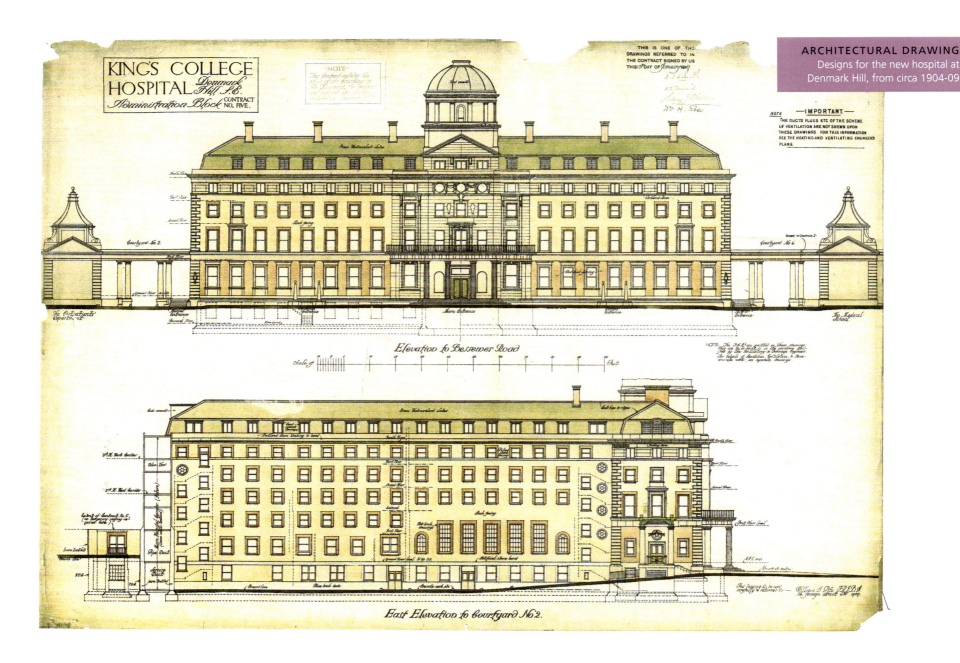

KING'S COLLEGE
HOSPITAL *Denmark Hill S.E.*
Administration Block CONTRACT NO. FIVE.

Elevation to Bessemer Road

East Elevation to Courtyard No 2.

ARCHITECTURAL DRAWING
Designs for the new hospital at
Denmark Hill, from circa 1904-09

PORTUGAL STREET

The old King's College Hospital on Portugal Street, photographed around 1910

1912 - FIRST INSTALMENT OF £50,000, BY AN ANONYMOUS DONOR

The largest cheque given towards the removal of the hospital to Denmark Hill

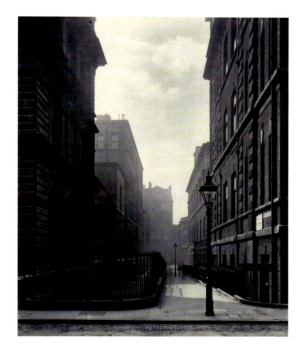

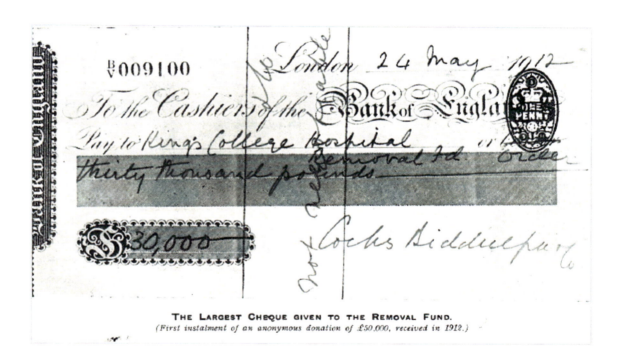

THE LARGEST CHEQUE GIVEN TO THE REMOVAL FUND.
(First instalment of an anonymous donation of £50,000, received in 1912.)

THE KING IN SOUTH LONDON

The *Westminster Gazette* describes King Edward VII's visit to lay the foundation stone of King's in Camberwell on July 20, 1909.

"The inhabitants of Camberwell gave the Royal Party an enthusiastic welcome. The whole route was profusely decorated… Some of the banners bore notable inscriptions. 'Welcome to his Majesty, the best friend of the poor and suffering,' ran one in the Walworth Road.

His Majesty in a clear voice read his reply [to the Hospital Committee's address]: 'It gives me great pleasure to come today to lay the foundation-stone of the new buildings of the hospital with which the Sovereign's name is connected… For many years King's College Hospital has ministered to the necessities and alleviated the sufferings of thousands of my subjects in the centre of this crowded Metropolis.

Your committee's decision to abandon the old buildings and to remove the scene of your labour to a poorer and more populous district where the need of a hospital was great… was a bold step. But I believe it was a wise and right one.'

Great crowds lined the streets in the vicinity of the hospital and loudly cheered their Majesties as they drove away."

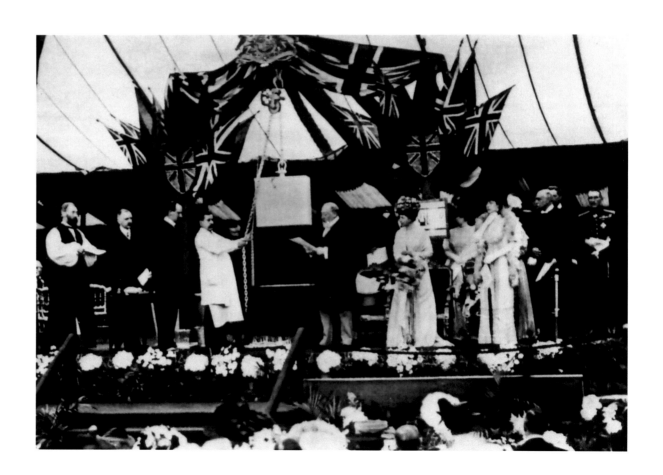

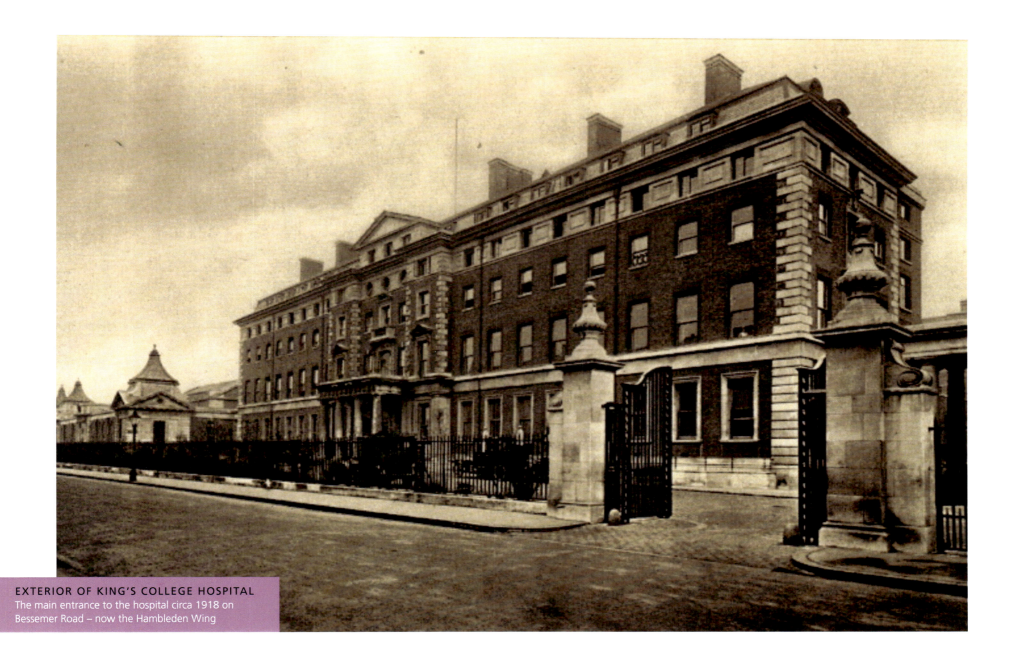

EXTERIOR OF KING'S COLLEGE HOSPITAL
The main entrance to the hospital circa 1918 on
Bessemer Road – now the Hambleden Wing

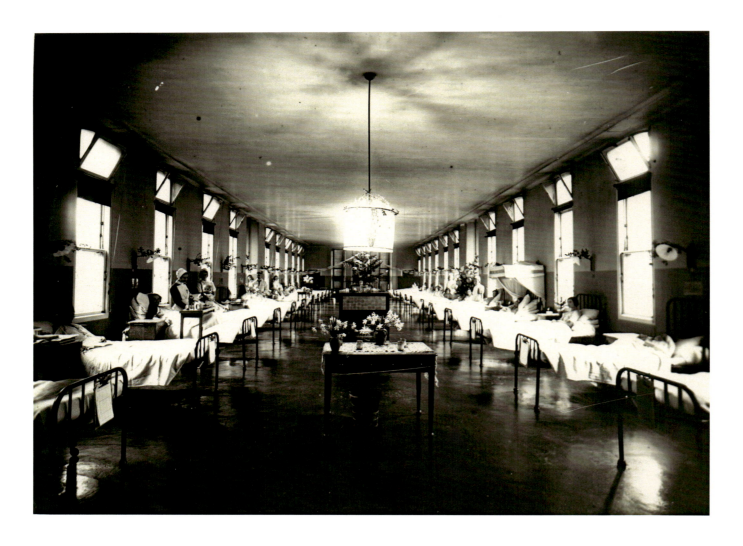

From its foundation in 1840 King's was a voluntary hospital; it depended on donations and private money. But in 1948 the NHS was created. In the next ten years the number of King's outpatients rose from 153,000 to 215,000 in the new era of comprehensive, universal healthcare.

FEMALE TWINING WARD
Photographed in 1930, the Twining Ward for female patients had no private cubicles or curtains

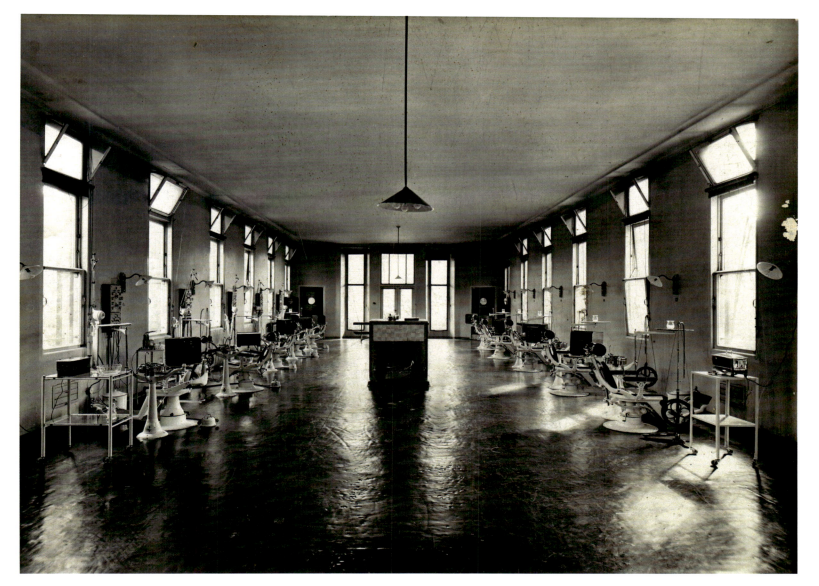

STUDENT DENTAL WARD
The Matthew Whiting Ward circa 1930, lined with dental chairs and used by students of the Dental School

Chapter 2

KING'S IN THE
TWO WORLD WARS

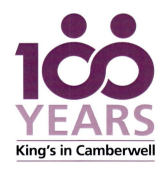

KING'S IN THE
TWO WORLD WARS

King's has served its country and survived two World Wars: the **Great War of 1914-18** and the **Second World War, 1939-45**. In both conflicts King's met the challenge of military emergencies and the needs of its civilian community. These were years of hardship for all, yet the war years also brought remarkable medical progress and cemented King's reputation for dedication and excellence

———

With the outbreak of the First World War in 1914, King's became the Fourth London General Military Hospital. Except for four wards and the casualty department, the hospital was cleared for military casualties. In three years, the hospital treated more than 75,000 wounded and injured soldiers. Tents and huts were constructed in Ruskin Park, opposite King's, to cope with the number of patients. A bridge was built over the Denmark Hill railway line that separated King's and the park to ease access.

The most serious cases from France were treated at King's. Trench foot – common among soldiers who served in the cold, damp trenches of France and Belgium – was treated with water baths and exercises. Cases of shell shock – psychological trauma caused by wartime experiences - were cared for on dedicated wards and quickly moved to special care homes.

When the hospital was returned to civilian use in 1919, King's was officially thanked for *"nobly and efficiently supplement[ing] the efforts of the Government in ministering the needs of the sick and wounded who were returned to the homeland for healing."*

Just 21 years later, the world was at war again. In the Second World War, King's served as an air raid casualty clearing station. In preparation, windows were taped to prevent flying glass, sandbags piled around hospital entrances, operating theatres moved to the hospital basement and arrangements made to move patients and beds from wards on the top floor to the basement during air raids.

Surgeon Harold Edwards was in charge of war preparations at King's. Just over a month after Prime Minister Neville Chamberlain declared war on September 3, 1939, Edwards wrote in his diary:

Tuesday October 10, 1939
"The grass is growing apace from the sandbags in front of King's. It gives the sandbags a detestable air of permanence – that air… with which we became so familiar in 1914-18."

King's was made ready to take in 200 patients at a moment's notice. The new basement operating theatre had four operating tables and a fridge

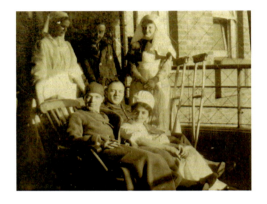

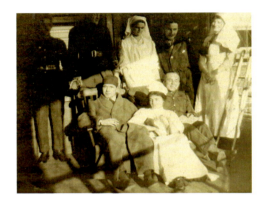

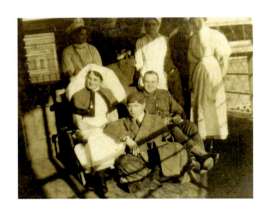

stocked with 40 litres of blood, of all types. Reception would direct patients to departments for major and minor dressings.

A large King's staff was ready for air raids, but for eight months Britain watched and waited – there were no air raids, just an uneasy calm. Civilian patients were still admitted for ordinary operations. But on September 7, 1940 the Blitz began in London; the Luftwaffe bombed the city for 57 consecutive nights. During the day, London's skies were full of dog fights between British Spitfires and German bombers.

Once assessed and stabilised at King's, air raid casualties were evacuated to hospitals in the suburbs, including Epsom and Leatherhead. Each morning, the matron reported the number of casualties admitted in air raids the night before. Remarkably, King's only suffered one direct hit in the entire 1939-1945 war when a small bomb landed on the entrance to the casualty department. However, St Matthew's Church opposite the hospital – now the site of the dental school – burned down in an air raid. Medical teaching

THE FOURTH LONDON GENERAL MILITARY HOSPITAL
First World War soldiers and military nurses photographed whilst King's was a military hospital

continued throughout the war, though King's students studied away from the hospital. Some of the hospital's consultants and surgeons also joined the forces, serving around the world from the Mediterranean to South East Asia.

If war drew the people of London together, with many civilians volunteering whatever help they could, both World Wars had another silver lining: medical progress. Physiotherapy, plastic surgery and rehabilitation were some of the areas that advanced at King's during First World War. The demands of World War II meanwhile brought more use of blood and intravenous infusions, greater use of aseptic (sterile) techniques and the discovery of sulfa drugs and antibiotics.

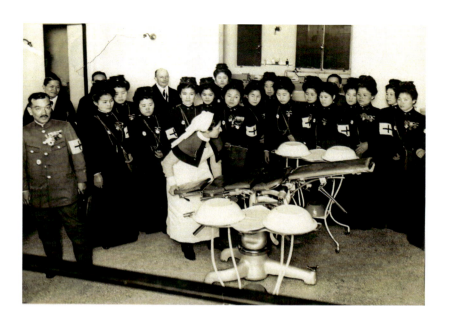

JAPANESE WAR VISIT
Between 1914 and 1915, the Japanese Ambassador visited King's with a group called the Japanese Air for Our Wounded. Here, a King's nurse demonstrates an operating table

MILITARY NURSES
Voluntary civilian nurses joined the existing King's nurses during the First World War

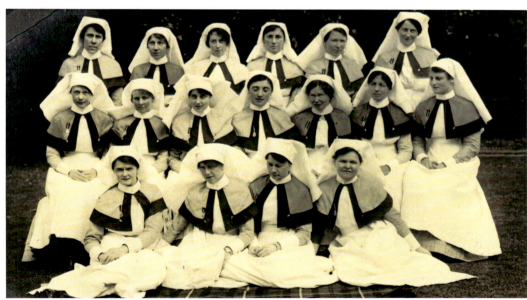

NURSES DURING THE WAR

Nurses' uniforms were shortened – to accommodate rationing.

Nurses also had their own rations and kept individual supplies of treats – butter, jam, sugar – on labelled shelves in the dining room.

Day nurses would sleep on bunks in the basement – rather like the staff in Prime Minister Churchill's own Cabinet War Rooms in Whitehall.

WARTIME
MEMORY

Annie Mary Esler, civilian nurse with the Red Cross Voluntary Aid Detachment (VAD) at King's, 1917-18, speaking to the Imperial War Museum

"I was in the operating theatre practically all the time I was at King's. It was busy, sterilising the theatre from one case to another because we had them streaming in all day. Amputations, abdominal operations, bullet wounds through their backs and spines – they were completely paralysed. That stuck in my memory.

There was a room they called the 'dirty room', leading off the theatre where they put all the [amputated] arms and legs – which sounds horrible – because there were a tremendous lot of amputations. But we had to sit in there and have our coffee, which wasn't very pleasant. I didn't find it upsetting; you were so busy you didn't notice these horrible things happening. One looks back on it now with absolute horror.

We used to go off duty at night almost crying we were so tired. We lived right up Denmark Hill in a big private house there; eight of us slept in the dormitory together. We had to trudge up this hill at night, often in pitch black, after coming off duty."

PEACETIME PET
King's nurses, matron - and dog - photographed between the wars

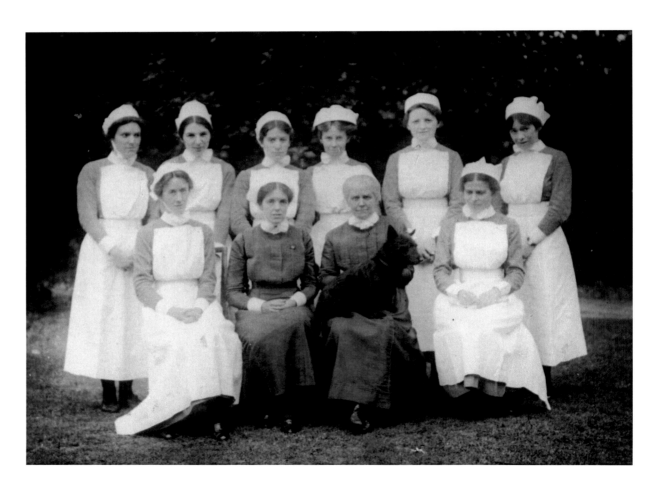

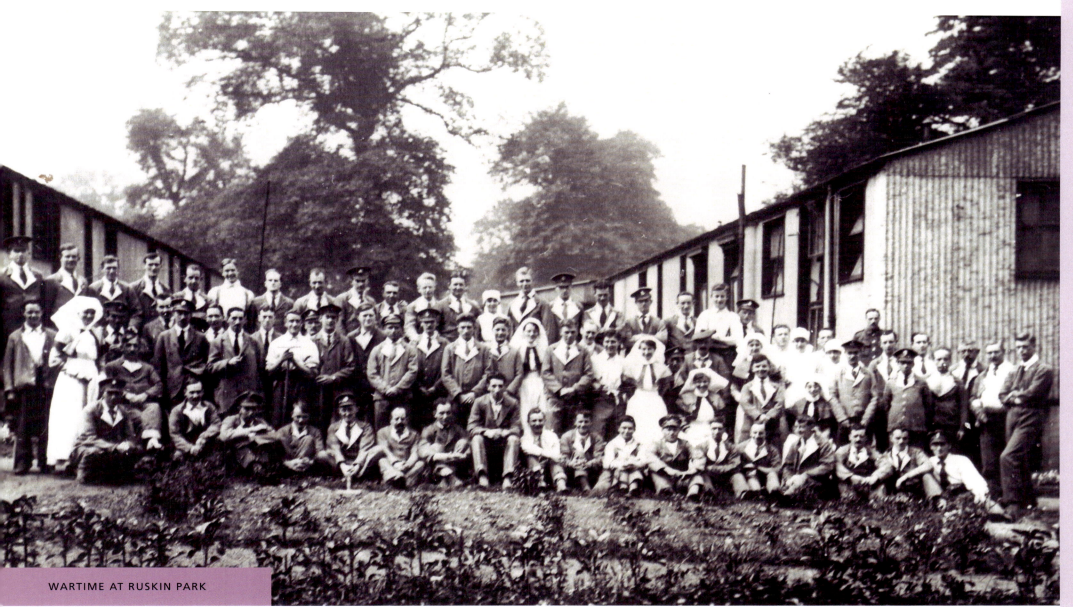

WARTIME AT RUSKIN PARK

RECUPERATION IN RUSKIN PARK
Wounded soldiers in invalid chairs being taken round the grounds at the Fourth London General Military Hospital © Imperial War Museum (Q 27814)

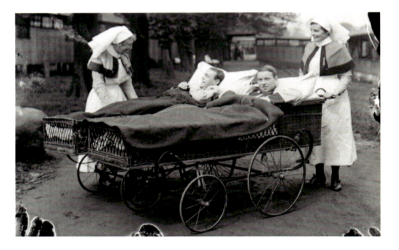

MAKESHIFT WARDS
"Open air" wards at the Fourth London General Military Hospital at Denmark Hill. Hospitals in England were used when pressure on the facilities in France became too great © Imperial War Museums (Q 27819)

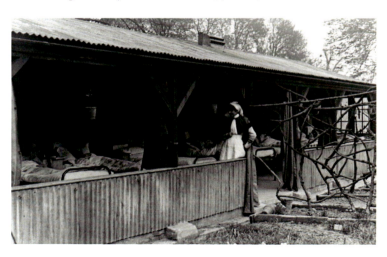

WARTIME EMERGENCY THEATRE
A basement operating theatre in around 1944. Surgery continued during blackouts, lit by oil lanterns

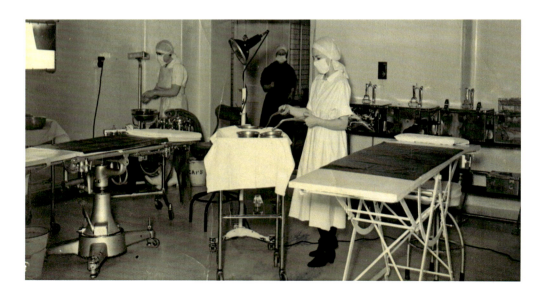

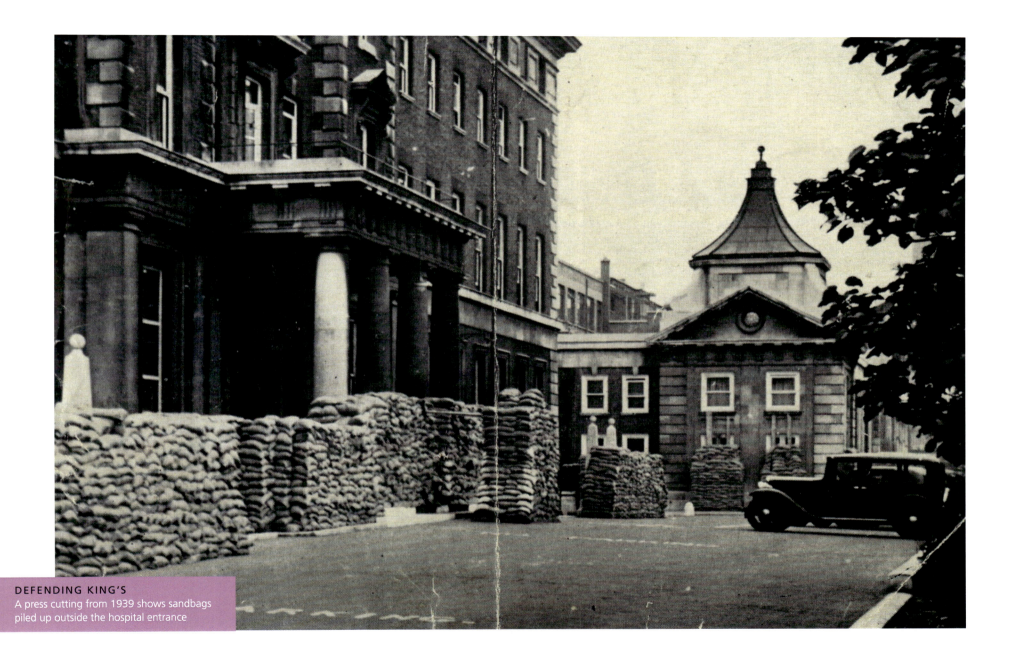

DEFENDING KING'S
A press cutting from 1939 shows sandbags
piled up outside the hospital entrance

Chapter 3

PATIENT AND STAFF LIFE
AT KING'S

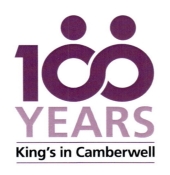

PATIENT AND STAFF LIFE
AT KING'S

One hundred years ago the brand new wards of King's had open coal-fires and a coal box at the door. A large iron bath was wheeled around to the beds – though it was so heavy, only the most privileged patients ever used it. Medication was brought to each ward in a wicker basket. **What was state of the art in 1913 seems archaic today.** King's life has changed dramatically

---

Decade by decade, life at King's has transformed for patients and staff alike. Patients received their first entertainment – wireless – in 1926, unveiled by the then Prime Minister Stanley Baldwin's wife. *The Spectator* magazine remarked: *"What a boon wireless is to the inmates of hospitals! Many patients too ill to read or talk, have energy enough to put on the head-phones."* By 1975, patients were tuning into Radio King's: *"Introducing new sounds on the pop scene, sweet, and occasionally classical music."*

Television arrived in King's paediatric wards in the 1950s but adults had to wait until 1968, when the *South London Observer* excitedly reported: *"Each day-room is equipped for television relay for all programmes including BBC2 colour."* But true luxury had arrived seven years earlier when patients no longer had to wake up for breakfast at 5:30am but at a leisurely 8am.

Today, children recovering from surgery on Princess Elizabeth Ward can play Nintendos, and a room designed specifically for teenage patients offers magazines, CDs and computers for their use. King's also has many family rooms, cafes and day rooms for patients, staff and visitors, while pictures brighten the corridors and wards. Many of these changes are funded by the Friends of King's College Hospital. Begun as the Ladies Association in 1917, it became the Friends in 1961 and includes the junior Kingfishers. The Friends provide a Trolley Service around the wards, and they have donated specialist medical equipment, bedside chairs and TVs for day rooms, wards and staff rooms. In 2012 the friends donated funds to help transform the Marjory Warren Ward which treats and cares for older people, many of whom will have dementia. It is a specially designed 'sensory' ward which provides a friendlier and more relaxing environment for patients. The ward was named after Dr Marjory Warren (1897 - 1960), a surgeon who pioneered specialist healthcare for older patients.

Life for nurses at King's has also changed radically. After getting jugs of beer with their dinner in 1918, nurses seemed to lurch backwards in the 1950s into strict regulations. Rules issued by Matron's office in 1957 state that nurses could *"entertain visitors to tea between 4pm and 5pm daily."* But only two guests were allowed at a time. Outdoor uniform comprised a navy overcoat *"which must always be buttoned"*, a beret *"worn over the*

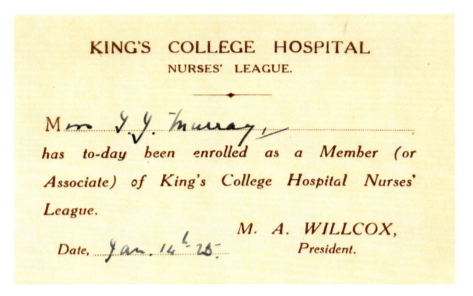

NURSES LEAGUE ENROLMENT CARD (ABOVE)
Formed in 1924, the Nurses League is a social network for nurses, past and present

TRAINING CERTIFICATE (RIGHT)
Nurse Grace Lizzie Buttard's certificate of nursing exams from 1911-14

left ear", black gloves and handbag. *"Nurses may wear outdoor uniform as far as Camberwell Green, but should never wear it in places of public entertainment. No nurse may smoke in outdoor uniform."*
King's prowess doesn't only lie within its hospital walls. In 1928 the inaugural King's College Hospital Medical School sports day saw a high standard of track and field, including a winning 4 minutes and 32 seconds in the mile race. By 1967, sports day had evolved to include an egg and spoon race – and a consultants' race.

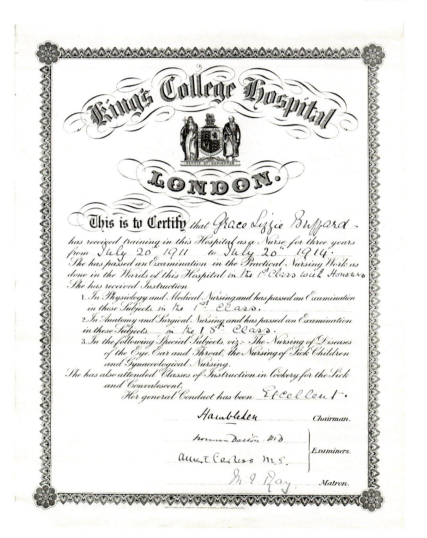

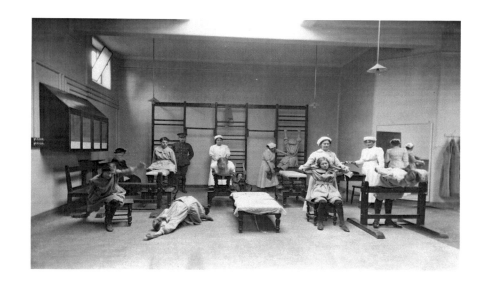
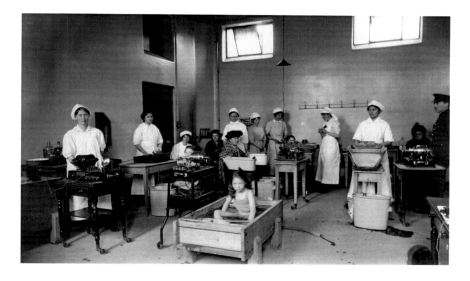
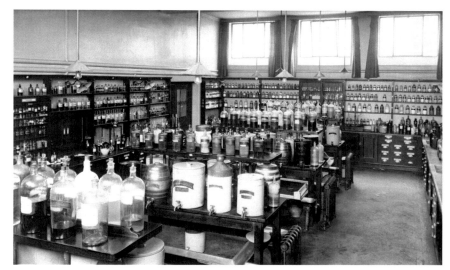
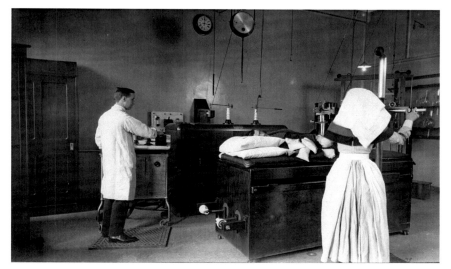

KING'S INTERIOR
Photographed between 1913 and 1929, working life in (clockwise from top left) the rather uncomfortable-looking gymnasium, the electrical department,
King's dispensary and the radiography department

OUTPATIENT INVITE
In 1915 women were invited to attend
Dr Charlton Briscoe's Wednesday clinic

WASHING NEWBORN BABIES
Nurses bathe newborn babies circa 1915. In
1974 midwifery, nursing and physiotherapy
moved to the newly opened Normanby College

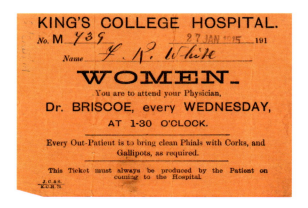

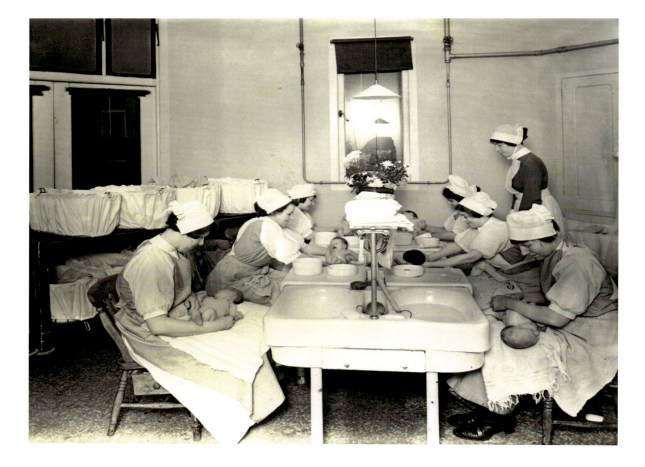

CHRISTMAS POSTCARD
The Todd Maternity Ward decorated for Christmas – with a tree just visible behind the desk – in about 1920

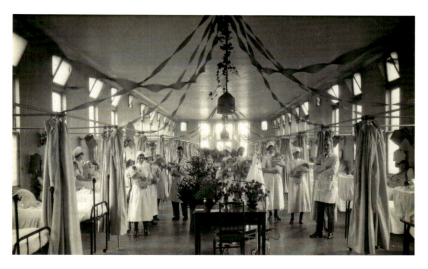

NURSES AT DINNER
A nursing dinner circa 1920, possibly in the nurses' recreational room. Nurses took turns to sit at Sister Matron's table

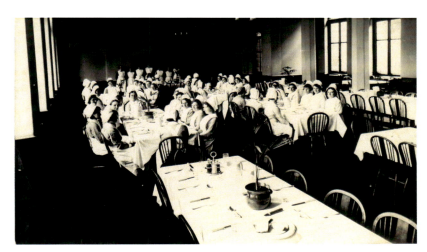

DOCTORS AND STUDENTS CELEBRATING
Patients look on as doctors and students carry a colleague on their shoulders in 1931, possibly celebrating a sporting success

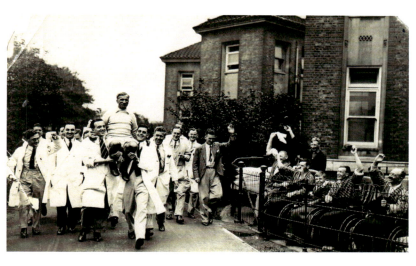

CHOIR PRACTICE
Never mind the medicine… nurses relax in the choir.

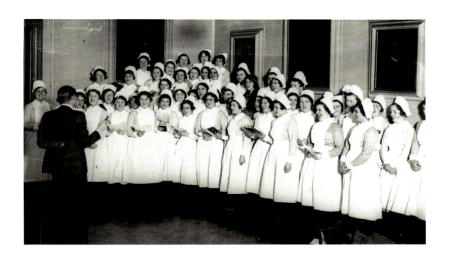

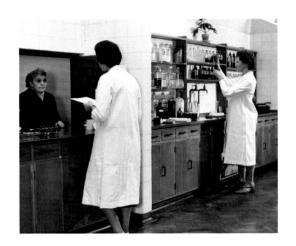

DISPENSARY
A patient waits for a prescription from the King's dispensary in 1959 (left)

NURSE TRAINING
Student nurses training to apply bandages, photographed (below and right) in around 1945

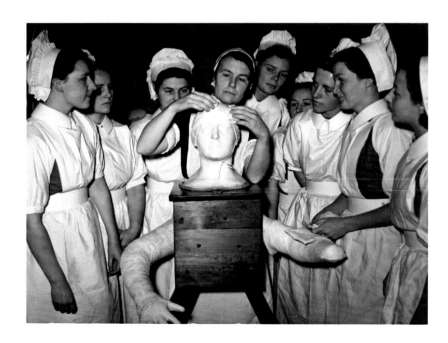

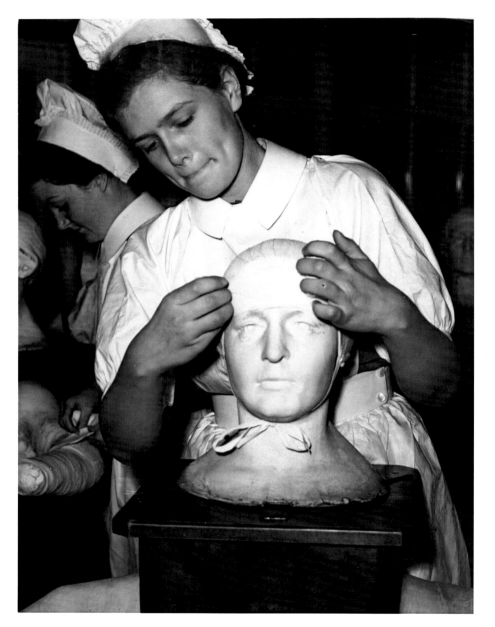

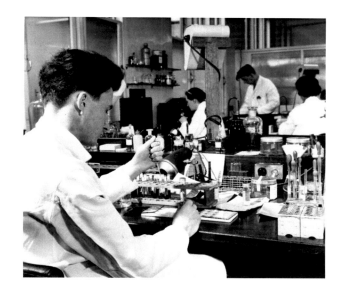
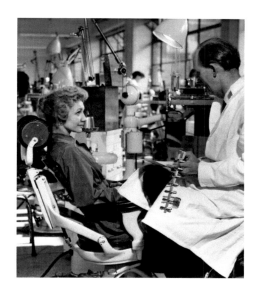
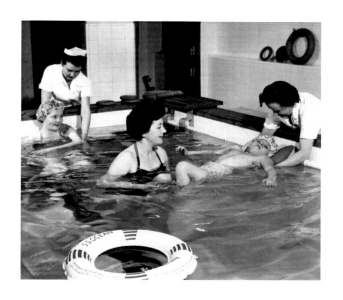

TREATMENTS

In 1959 *Country Life* magazine photographed the bacteriology lab, dental ward, physiotherapy pool, wards and operating theatre. The X-ray photo dates from 1980 (bottom middle)

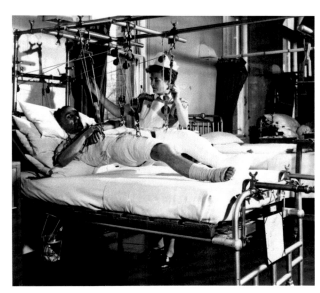
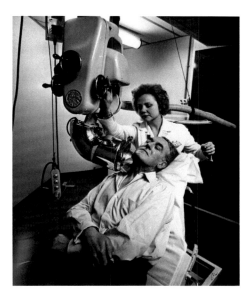
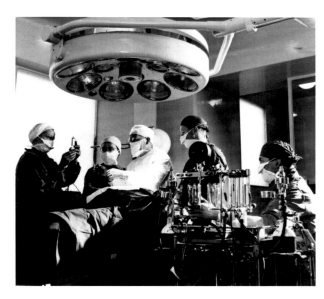

A LIFETIME AT KING'S

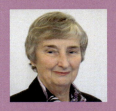

Rowenna Hughes

Rowenna Hughes has had a 45-year association with King's. Originally a paediatric physiotherapist, she joined the board of governors in 2006 and has been Chair of the Friends of King's for five years

"When I was six or seven I was a Kingfisher – I had a badge and a collection box. Then I became a Friend. The Friends are here to fundraise for the benefit of staff and patients. We've given the staff fridges, microwaves, kettles, newly decorated dayrooms to sit in and relax. Last year we received a legacy and created the Rosa Davis sensory room in the Marjory Warren Ward. It looks lovely.

The wards have changed unbelievably since the 1960s; they're cleaner and much brighter. I used to be petrified of Matron. She marched around the wards checking everything was clean and tidy. We had to have the bed wheels facing the right way, the pillows correct, the sheets just so regardless of whether the patient was cold or hot. The whole atmosphere of the wards is more homely these days."

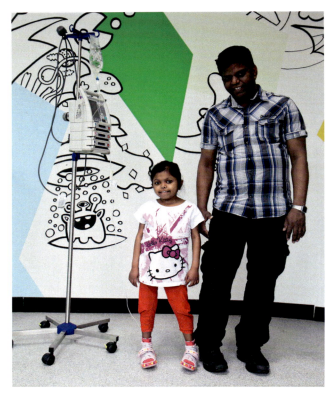

HOSPITAL LIFE - PRESENT DAY

In 1961 a King's committee on noise investigated the efficacy of soundproof hoods for snoring patients.

In 1967 stilettos were banned in the new Dental School – the heels were damaging the new floors.

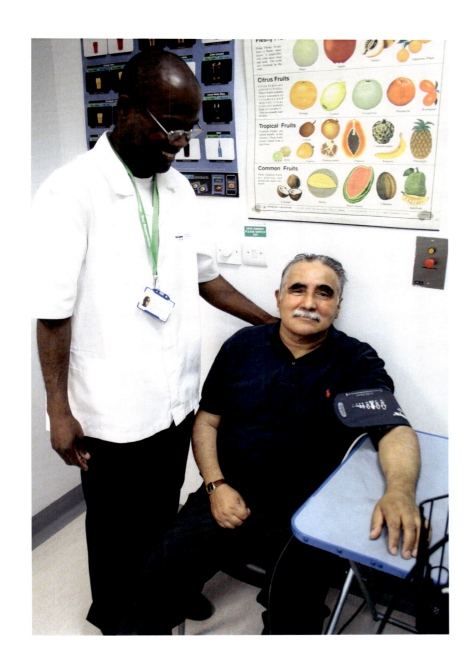

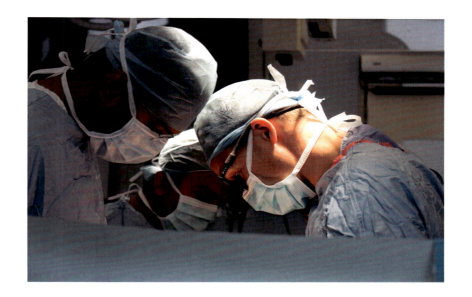

HOSPITAL LIFE - PRESENT DAY

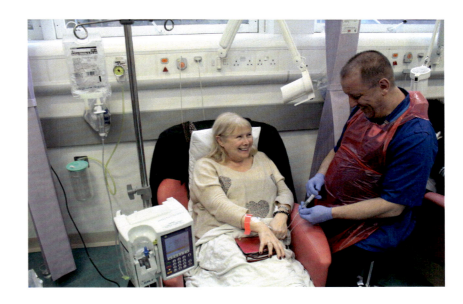

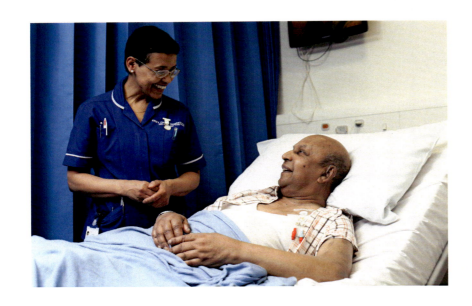

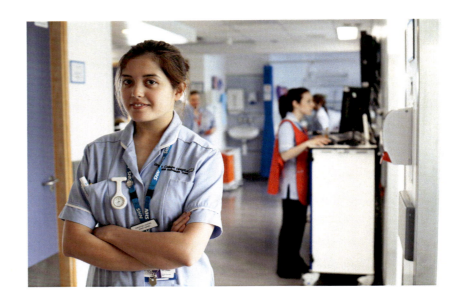

HOSPITAL LIFE - PRESENT DAY

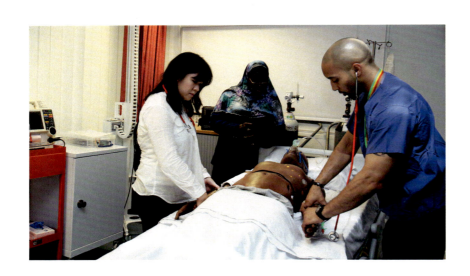

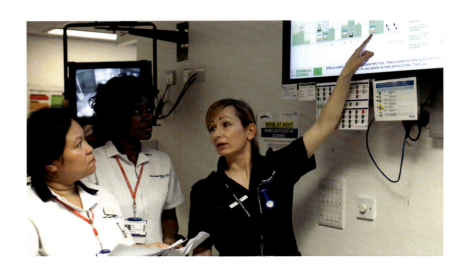

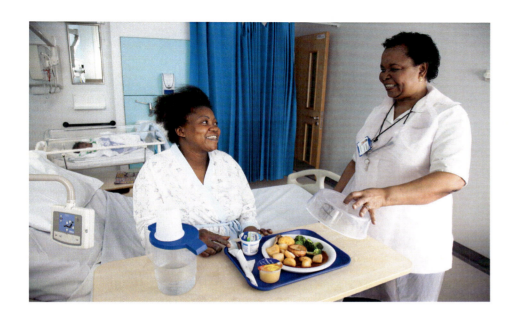

HOSPITAL LIFE - PRESENT DAY

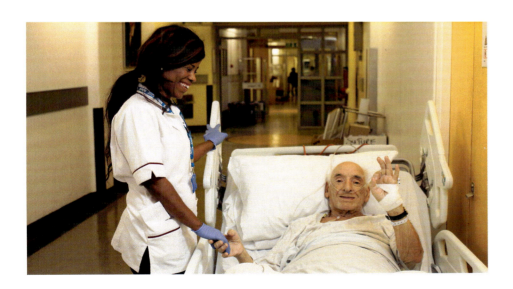

A KING'S PERSON

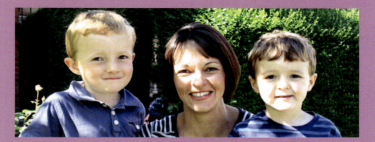

Sharlene Greenwood was a physiotherapy student at King's, where she met her husband Jim. Her two sons were born at King's – and so was their grandfather! Sharlene is now lead Renal Physiotherapist at King's

"I first came to King's on a student physiotherapy placement – it was amazing because you would see surgery and rehab. I returned as a junior because the physiotherapy department was really dynamic. Professionally, King's is a great place to work and do research. Our renal department is one of the best in the country and the first to develop renal exercise clinically. We've just been awarded a £2.1m grant to do a trial of exercise while on dialysis.

I've never left because I've always had an opportunity to further myself here. I'm a King's person through and through.

We've had both of our sons at King's: Harry, five, was born on the maternity ward and Lawrie, four, was born with the King's home birth service. Harry has also been a patient under the paediatric orthopaedic service, and the care was absolutely fantastic. It made me proud to be part of King's."

Chapter 4

KING'S IN
ITS COMMUNITY

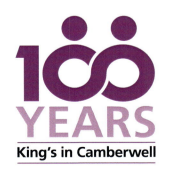

KING'S IN
ITS COMMUNITY

King's is unusual in that it is a **major London teaching hospital**, but is also rooted in **a diverse local community**. For 100 years it has met the changing health needs of **Camberwell, Brixton and Peckham** with pioneering treatment and medical expertise. Today, King's inspires great **affection and pride in its community** – and **some extraordinary fundraising**

King's had barely opened its doors in Denmark Hill when medics had to contend with a flu epidemic. TH Whittington, a doctor who worked for 74 years at King's, spoke of the 1918-19 emergency: *"It was terrible. People coming back from the war having been away from their families all those years, only to die in this country."* King's has continued to serve the community's health needs ever since. From cholera in the late 19th century, to tuberculosis in the 1920s, to sickle cell disease today, King's has met the challenge.

In such ethnically and economically diverse area as Lambeth and Southwark, King's supports a population with above average rates of cardiovascular disease, HIV and teenage pregnancy. Meanwhile, male life expectancy remains below the national average. As a Major Trauma Centre, King's is also working with police and community groups to educate its local population about knife and gun crime, and to prevent injury.

But the community around King's has an incredible advantage: a world-leading research facility on its doorstep offering the newest treatments to many patients. Love, pride and respect clearly exist between the community and King's. Eight hundred volunteers from schools and local community organisations now help around the hospital. They visit wards, spend time with patients, welcome and direct visitors at the main entrances. Half of these volunteers are under 25 years old.

In fact, the community has long returned help to King's. *"I was told many stories of the generosity of the less well-off section of the community,"* remarked a writer from *The Spectator* magazine, when he visited King's in 1929. *"Five women in domestic service… contributed out of their small wages sufficient to pay for a bed."* And in 1937, when the hospital faced a funding crisis, the *Camberwell and Peckham Times* ran a campaign encouraging readers to fundraise. One man had an ingenious scheme. On May 12, 1937, the day of George VI's coronation, he posted himself nine envelopes, each marked with three stamps: the heads of George V, Edward VIII, George VI – the past, abdicating and new Kings. *"If any of our readers are philatelists and would like to secure one of these souvenirs and at the same time help King's they are invited to make an offer,"* announced the paper.

1913   2013

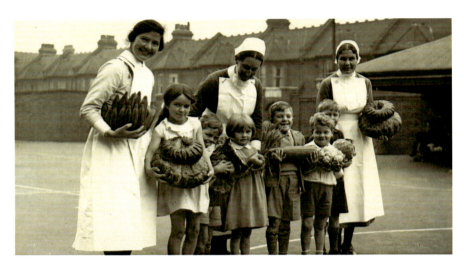

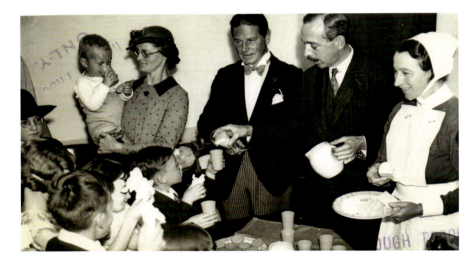

Since 2011, the staff of King's Emergency Department (ED) have taken centre stage in Channel 4's award-winning documentary series *24 Hours in A&E*. This is the channel's largest ever documentary series, watched by three million people every week and now broadcast to almost 100 countries worldwide. In 2013 the series was nominated for a British Academy of Film and Television Arts (BAFTA) Award in the Factual Series category.

King's also appeared on television 50 years ago in a BBC documentary called *They Made History: Joseph Lister,* about the pioneer of antiseptic surgery, Dr Joseph Lister.

And in 2009, King's neurosurgeon Nicholas Thomas performed a pituitary tumour removal live on Channel 4 as part of The Operation: *Surgery Live* series. The work that makes the King's local community so proud is reaching audiences many miles away.

HARVEST FESTIVAL (LEFT)
King's nurses with local children circa 1920, excited about harvest festival

TEA PARTY AT KING'S (RIGHT)
A community tea party for children visiting King's in 1936, possibly organised by the Nurses League

In 1929 *The Spectator* magazine suggested an advertising slogan to appear on the front of King's: "Fill up here with health!"

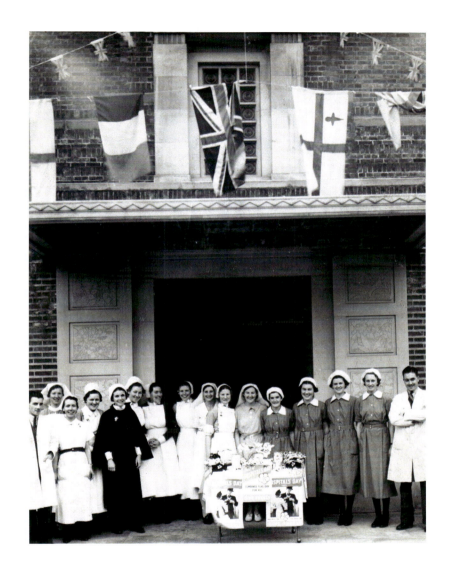

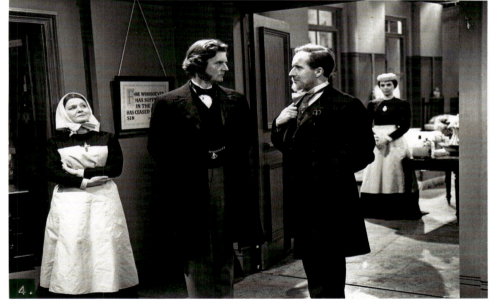

FLAG DAY
Nurses sell flags to raise money for
King's on Hospital Day in 1938

KING'S ON TV
Among King's earliest appearances on TV was the BBC's *They Made History:*
Joseph Lister, a dramatisation of Lister's story in 1960

OUR CHANCE
TO GIVE BACK

Fundraisers explain why they are committed to King's

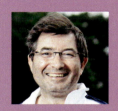

Andy Strachan

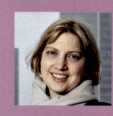

Sara Pedre

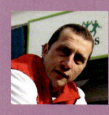

Steve Huckle

Andy Strachan had a liver transplant at King's in 2010. *"I fundraise for King's because I'm trying to give something back. Anything helps. It's about those little extras that make life easier for people. Money I've raised has bought laptops for patients. TV is OK but in this day and age it really helps if you can get emails, look at the news. Fundraising doesn't take a lot of time and you get a lot out of it."*

Sara Pedre developed a large, cancerous lesion on her liver and had the transplant just three months after her diagnosis. Now she leads a normal life again and donates to King's every month. *"I give because I owe everything to them. I feel so incredibly blessed to be under their care. I'd like others who have suffered, or who are suffering now, to benefit from the kind of treatment that I had."*

Steve Huckle's daughter Tara was diagnosed with a brain tumour at just a year old. She was cared for by Thomas Cook Children's Critical Care Centre and Lion Ward. Steve has completed two cycling challenges for King's: from Land's End to John O'Groats and from London to Nice. *"Those challenges were about thanking King's and also overcoming something difficult, just like Tara had to. They were a means for me to understand, in a small way, some of what Tara has had to go through."*

You can find out more about donating to King's at: www.togetherwecan.org.uk/kings-college-hospital

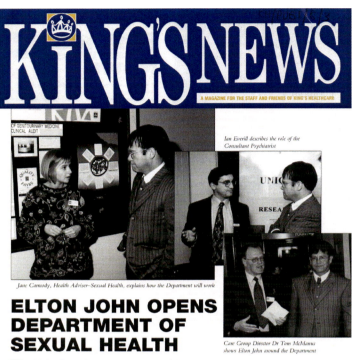

THE ROCKET MAN AT KING'S (ABOVE)

Elton John opened the department of sexual health at King's in 1993, reported in *King's News*, the staff and friends' magazine. King's liver department was the first in the UK, in the mid 1990s, to transplant patients with HIV and liver disease – originally believed impossible with a weakened immune system

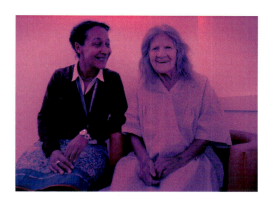

LEFT
Emma Ouldred, Memory Clinic Sister/Dementia Nurse Specialist in Department of Clinical Gerontology with a patient in the sensory room

BOTTOM LEFT
Lisa de Jonge, Matron (Donne, Marjory Warren and Byron Wards), with a patient

BELOW
Yamu Njie, Ward Manager, with a patient

MARJORY WARREN WARD - ROSA DAVIS SENSORY ROOM
The Marjory Warren Ward has 30 beds and is part of the Health and Ageing Unit. It is a specially designed 'sensory' ward which provides a friendlier and more relaxing environment for patients. The ward is named after Dr Marjory Warren (1897-1960), a surgeon who pioneered specialist healthcare for elderly patients

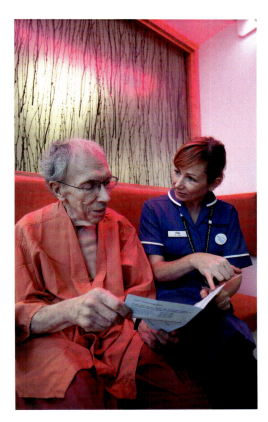

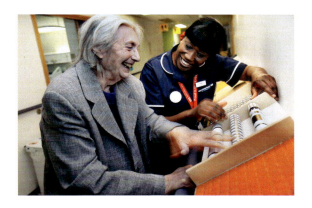

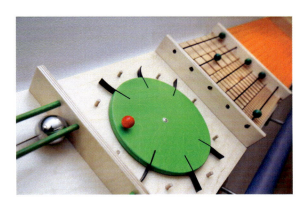

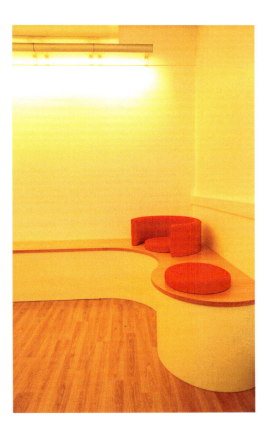

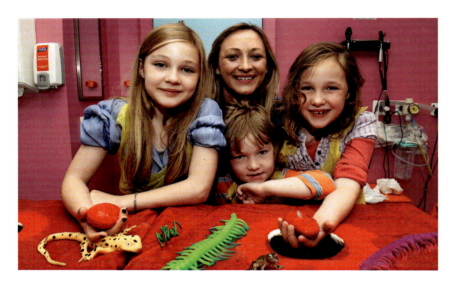

FRIENDS OF KING'S COLLEGE HOSPITAL
The friends provide a trolley service around the wards, and fundraise to help the hospital, staff and patients

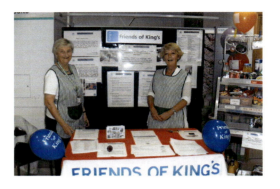

KING'S OPEN DAY (ABOVE AND BELOW)
The annual King's open cay gives the community a look at hospital life and kids a chance to operate

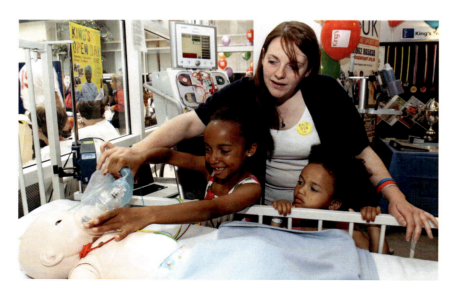

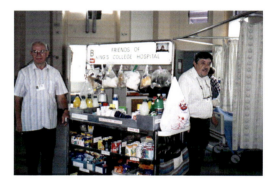

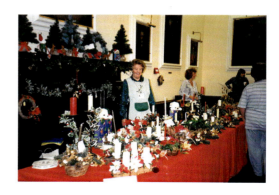

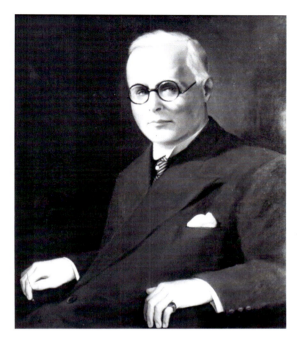

PERCY LANE OLIVER - BLOOD TRANSFUSION
From the first voluntary blood donation in 1921 Percy Lane Oliver's vision has grown to 107 million blood donations globally in 2013

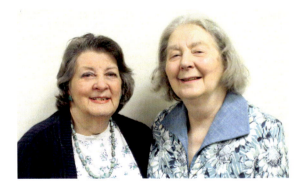

GRANDDAUGHTERS OF PERCY LANE OLIVER
Marion Cayless and her sister Helen Hardy (right)

A COMMUNITY PIONEER

In 1921, Camberwell Red Cross member and council book-keeper Percy Lane Oliver received a phone call from King's; they needed a blood donor. Oliver persuaded four friends to give blood and so began the world's first voluntary blood donor service, which Oliver ran from his home in Peckham and then Camberwell until he died in 1944. His granddaughters Helen Hardy, 82, and Marion Cayless, 77, share a remarkable story

Marion: Two rooms downstairs in the house were devoted to the blood service; we lived upstairs.

Helen: Grandpa had a vast filing cabinet with details of every donor and an map at home marked with people's addresses and all the hospitals. The phone could go morning, noon and night.

Marion: We always had to be quiet in the morning because grandpa didn't get up very early after being on duty all night. Hospitals would ring and ask for a particular blood group and he would go through the card index and find a suitable person. They'd go to the hospital to give the blood; it went from arm to arm because you couldn't store blood then. But you could store blood plasma – that's why we had a fridge. Not many people had a fridge.

Helen: We didn't ask an awful lot about the service. It was just something that went on at home. I don't know where he got the idea; it wasn't like one of these scientific things where several people think of the same thing at the same time. Grandpa was very gregarious and this was his baby so he publicised it as much as possible.

Marion: Our grandma thought he was wonderful. She was one of the first to give blood. She was being a good wife.

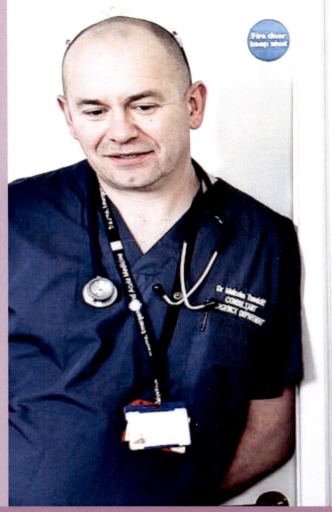

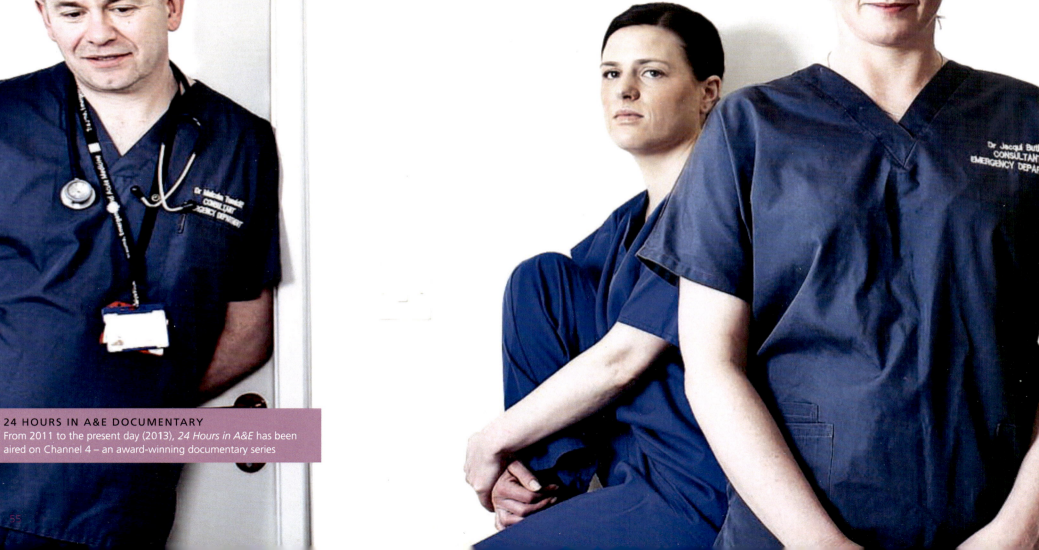

24 HOURS IN A&E

24 HOURS IN A&E DOCUMENTARY
From 2011 to the present day (2013), *24 Hours in A&E* has been aired on Channel 4 – an award-winning documentary series

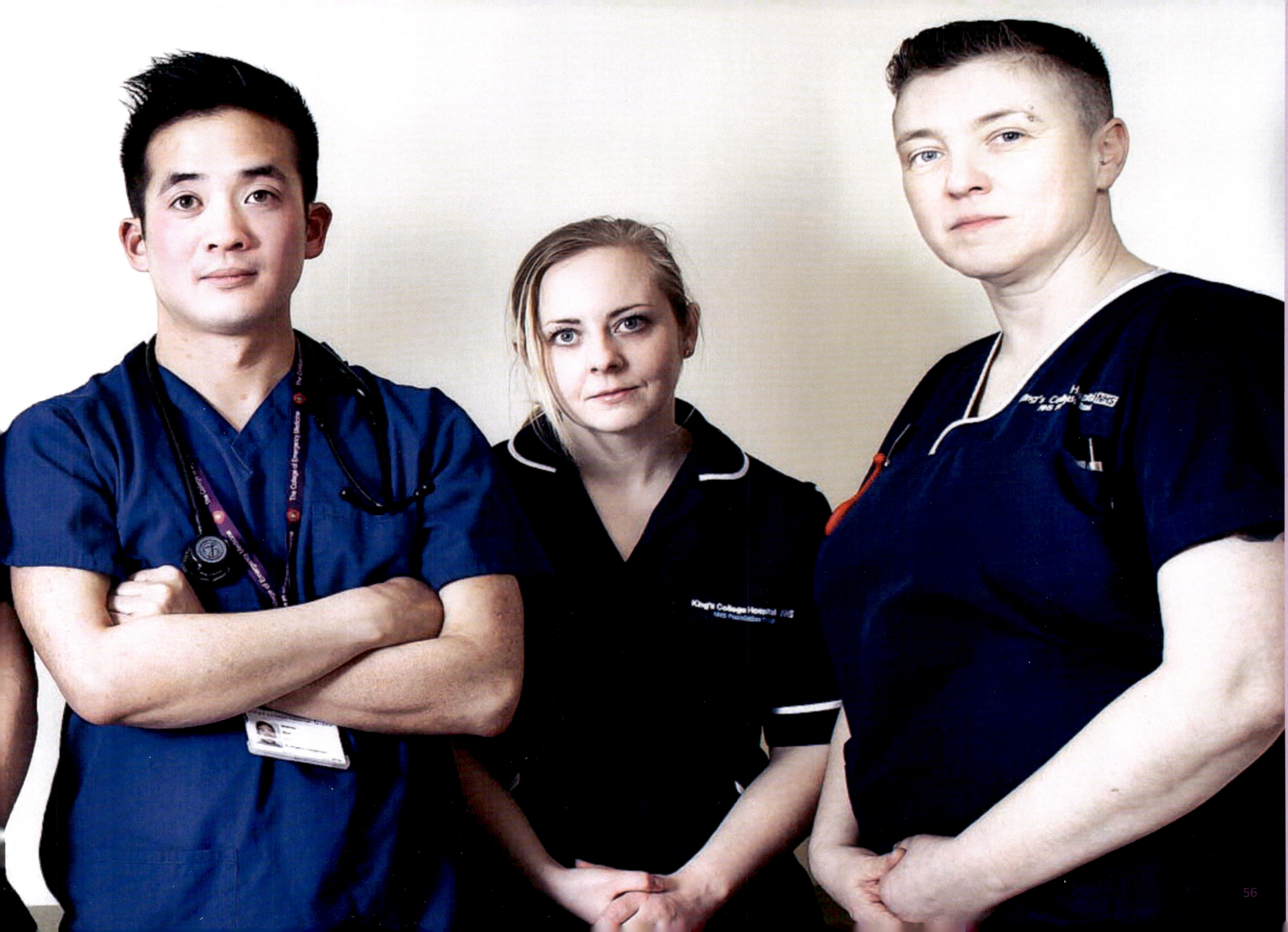
King's College Hospital NHS

Chapter 5

A CENTURY OF EXPANSION
AND MODERNISATION

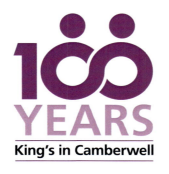

A CENTURY OF EXPANSION
AND MODERNISATION

From **300 beds** and just four operating theatres to **900 beds**, **26 operating theatres** and more than **7000 staff**, King's has mushroomed in its 100 years at Denmark Hill. In this story of transformation, major new buildings have a place alongside tiny new labs that produce the first shoots of life-changing medical research

In a century, the King's campus at Denmark Hill has expanded from a single new building to 15 buildings and wings containing wards, a children's hospital, specialist centres and departments – most of them squeezed inside a rectangle formed by Denmark Hill, Ruskin Park, Coldharbour Lane and Northlands Street. Among the major openings was a dental school in 1923. Dental chairs lined the walls of the Matthew Whiting Ward where you could get a filling for 1 shilling (around £1.50 today).

A sparkling new dental school was completed 43 years later; nicknamed Cocker's Castle after the chair of dentistry Ralph Cocker, it could take 50 students a year and treat 300 patients a day. At the same time, the New Ward Block was being completed beside Ruskin Park. This flagship ten storey building now known as the Ruskin Wing, opened in 1968 at an estimated cost of £1,350,000 (around £20m today). It had 168 beds, a maternity unit, special care baby units and clinics for obstetrics, gynaecology and infertility.

The seeds of world-leading research in liver transplantation were sown in the 1970s when a lab complex was built above Todd Ward. Research in the liver

unit really flourished in 1979 when the Sheik Zaid Centre opened. Today, most outpatients arrive at the Golden Jubilee Wing, the most recent major addition to King's in 2002. It is the largest hospital wing at King's College Hospital, patients come here for orthopaedics, X-rays, the world-famous Harris Birthright Centre, physiotherapy, maternity and more. Costing £75m, the front of the Golden Jubilee Wing is a four storey-high, striking glazed curve that floods the building with natural light.

Modernisation has steadily transformed King's in line with medical breakthroughs, local needs and medical passions of the time. In October 1968 the *South London Observer* reported that *"space-age treatment"* had arrived at King's. In fact it was a system of bedside buzzers allowing patients to call nurses.

And among the more peculiar openings was the Sunlight Department, the height of medical fashion in the 1920s when ultra-violet light was believed to cure TB and rickets. *The Spectator* magazine visited King's in 1929 and witnessed the department in action: *"… rays of what is in effect artificial*

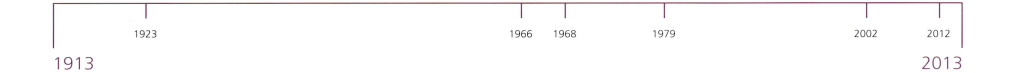

1923   1966   1968   1979   2002   2012

1913   2013

sunlight… pour from a mercury vapour lamp of dazzling brightness, and the patients who are receiving treatment sit in a circle about the lamp, exposing their bodies to the beams."

One King's area that has seen massive modernisation is the Emergency Department (ED), which now sees more than 130,000 patients a year. King's is one of only four Major Trauma Centres in London and also a Hyper Acute Stroke Unit. In 2012 a revolutionary new piece of kit arrived in the ED: a King's charity funded CT scanner, which takes detailed images of internal organs, blood vessels, bones and tumours. Patients with life-threatening injuries come straight to the CT scanner from an air or road ambulance. In the next few years, King's will improve its Major Trauma service further still with a new helipad and Critical Care Unit.

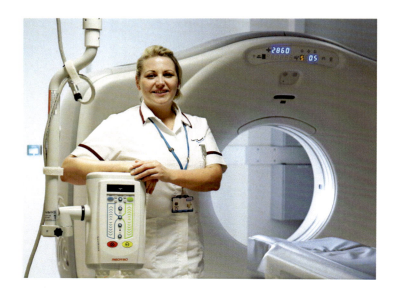

CT SCANNER
Kara Hollings, Trauma and Ortho Superintendent Radiographer in Radiology, with the new CT Scanner in 2012 – vital for specialist stroke and trauma care

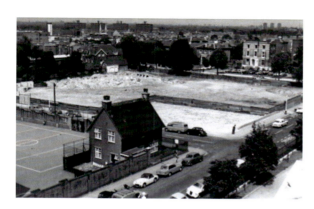

BEFORE
The new site of the Dental
Hospital on Bessemer Road
in 1962

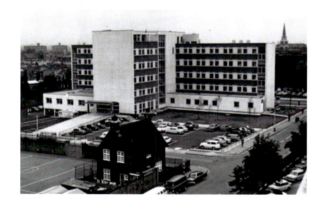

DENTAL WARD - AFTER
It opened in 1966, with labs,
phantom head rooms and
lecture theatres

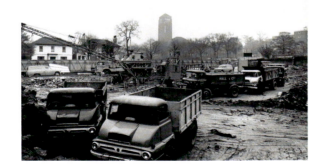

NEW WARD CONSTRUCTION
The ground is cleared for building
the Ruskin Wing in 1965

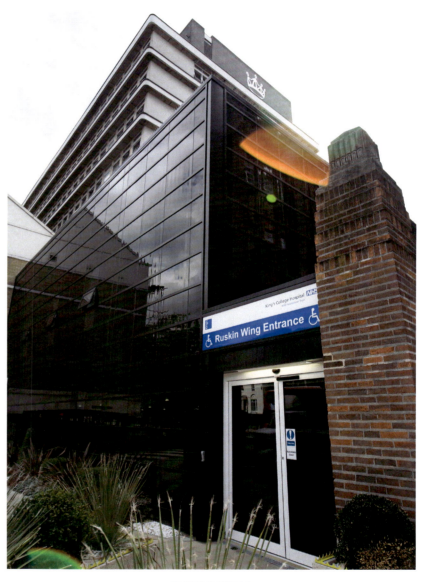

RUSKIN WING
Ruskin Wing today

WHAT IS IT DOING HERE?

King's Gazette, the staff magazine in 1972, discusses the arrival of the hospital's first computer system

"In 1969 the body of the beast arrived and settled in a new air-conditioned building. Since then its tentacles have been seen creeping though the fabric of the hospital… where treating it with reverence, amusement or disdain, everyone from the highest Professor to the lowest student spent countless hours feeding and studying it.

By 1972, the computer was used in two wards, haematology and admissions – where it was abandoned after two weeks having caused waiting list chaos.

Communication is achieved through VDUs (Visual Display Units) which consist of a small television screen (on which information from the computer, or a proposed message to it, is displayed) and a typewriter keyboard by which the information is put in… It is a good hour's work 'putting the patient on the computer' and so it is understandably unpopular with the housemen who were fully occupied beforehand. So far very little useful work is being done by the computer."

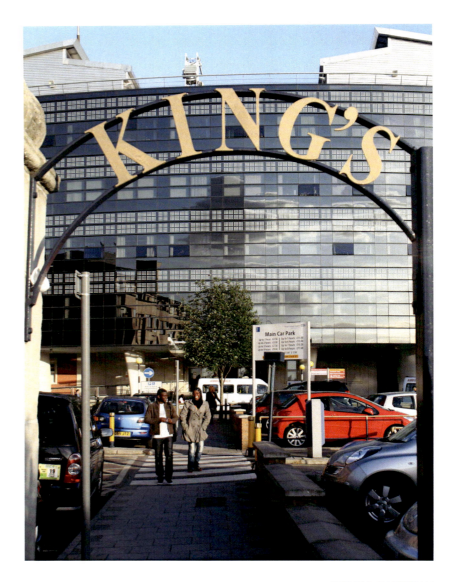

KING'S GATEWAY
The view from Caldecot Road, towards the Golden Jubilee Wing

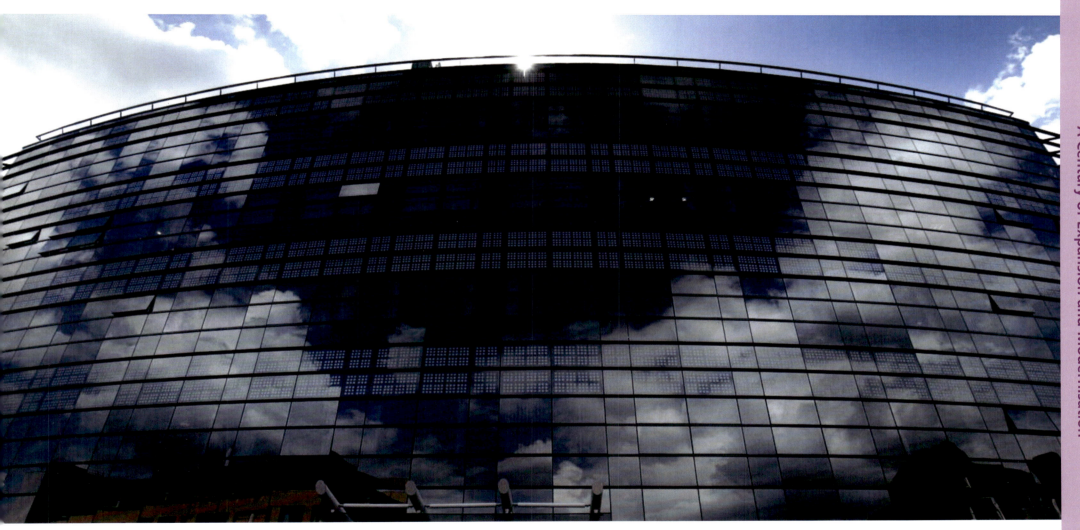

GOLDEN JUBILEE WING

In 2002 the Golden Jubilee Wing was completed – to date, the biggest addition to King's since 1913. It hosts outpatient clinics and wards, orthopaedics and the Harris Birthright Centre

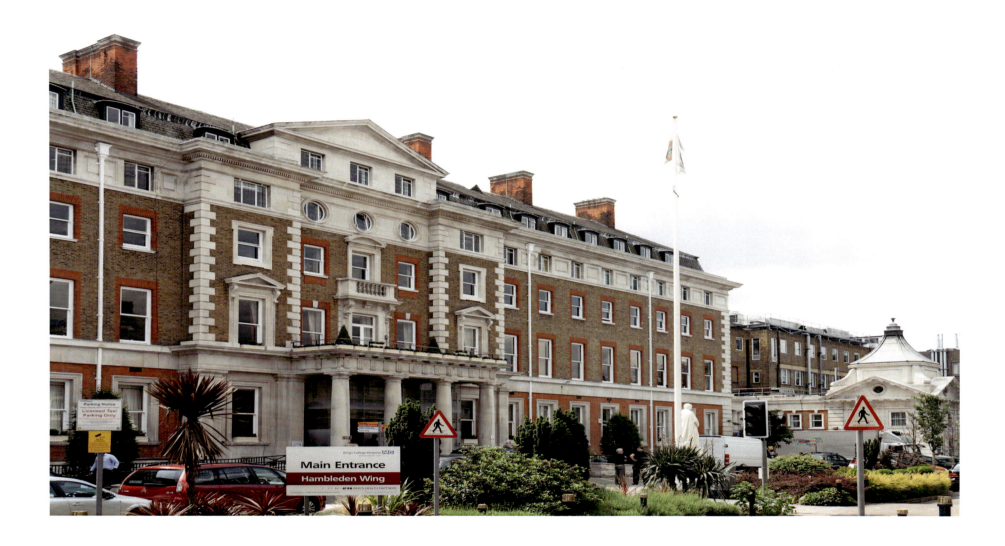

HAMBLEDEN WING
The original 1913 hospital building in 2013 with a statue of Robert Bentley Todd, the first Dean of King's, in front.
Behind the original entrance, Hambleden houses various clinical and administrative departments

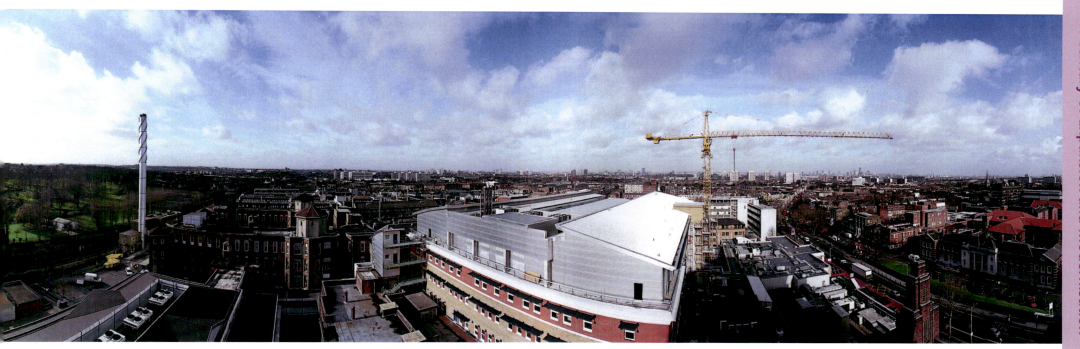

PANORAMIC VIEW OF KING'S

The panorama of the King's campus shows Denmark Hill to the right, with the tower of the 1930s Guthrie Wing for private and international patients just visible (bottom right corner). Ruskin Park is to the left. Cranes are a common sight at King's as the site is constantly updated. The campus is set to expand again soon with a new helipad and Critical Care Unit to improve King's facilities as a Major Trauma Centre

Chapter 6

A CENTURY OF
MEDICAL FIRSTS AT KING'S

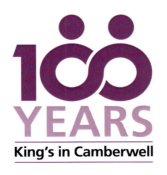

A CENTURY OF
MEDICAL FIRSTS AT KING'S

Pioneers of the **first bone marrow transplant in the UK**, the **first living related donor liver transplant in the UK**, and the **screening test for Down's Syndrome** now used throughout the world – the roll-call of King's medical firsts is outstanding. Thanks to its research ethos, **King's discoveries have saved and improved the lives** of its local population and patients who come to the hospital from around the world

The distinguished line of King's medical firsts begins in the 19th century with surgeon Joseph Lister. Rejected by many in the medical establishment, Lister was welcomed by King's as Professor of Clinical Surgery in 1877, where he perfected his technique of antiseptic surgery using sterilising carbolic spray.

"I wish germs were as obvious as green paint," Lister once said, as he turned the tide towards aseptic surgery. With his discovery, surgery was no longer (quite) the death-defying exercise it had been. Lister blew wide open the possibilities of surgery and paved the way for the life-changing operations performed today.

Fast forward to between the World Wars and diabetes care was revolutionised at King's. When doctor Robin Lawrence, 28, was diagnosed with the condition, he experimented on himself with a brand new treatment discovered in 1922: insulin. Lawrence set up a diabetic clinic at King's and in 1934 founded the Diabetic Association with *War of the Worlds* author H G Wells. Single-minded and devoted to his patients, by all accounts he was quite a character, signing off letters with 'Lorenzo il Magnifico'. Today, diabetic patients travel from around the UK to one of the world's first diabetic foot clinics, founded in 1981 by Professor Mike Edmonds, who has pioneered treatment that avoids the need for amputation.

Paediatrics remains another King's strength ever since Eric Stroud championed excellent healthcare for the deprived children of Camberwell in the 1960s. He transformed a small department into the Variety Children's Hospital, opened in 1985. King's paediatrics has pioneered specialist care for children with liver problems and sickle cell disease. And in 2010 a six-year-old boy at King's became the world's first patient to have a heart operation using MRI scan imaging instead of X-rays – saving the child from exposure to radiation.

In 1984 Sir James Black joined the Rayne Institute at King's as Professor of Analytical Pharmacology. Four years later he won the Nobel Prize in Medicine for developing beta blockers for treating heart disease, and anti-ulcer drugs. The James Black Foundation – a research centre – opened at Denmark Hill in 2007.

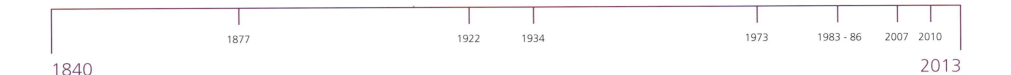

In neurology, King's not only treats patients with major head trauma but is known for its neurcsurgery firsts, and as a specialist centre for epilepsy and movement disorders. In 2013 the National Parkinson Foundation designated King's a centre of excellence for integrating care and research – one of only two centres in the UK.

In cardiology King's is part of the UK's largest aortic valve replacement programme; this new minimally invasive, keyhole procedure has the potential to help thousands of high-risk patients with artificial heart valves, without undergoing surgery.

In 1831, when anatomical specimens were in great demand, two men sold the corpse of a young Italian boy to King's College anatomical department. The boy had only recently been seen alive so the department called the Bow Street Runners (police officers). The two men were tried for murder and executed; one of the men's bodies was also kept by King's for dissection.

JOSEPH LISTER
Sterile surgery pioneer Lister at King's in 1890. He was considered a maverick by many, including medical journal The Lancet, in 1875: *"Few place faith in Lister's theory or carry out his practice – some have tried it, but they give it up for the weariness of the details."*

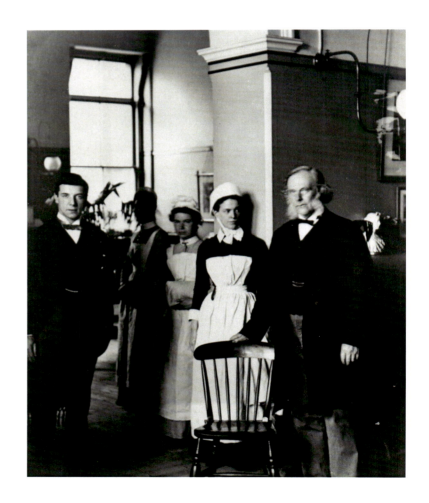

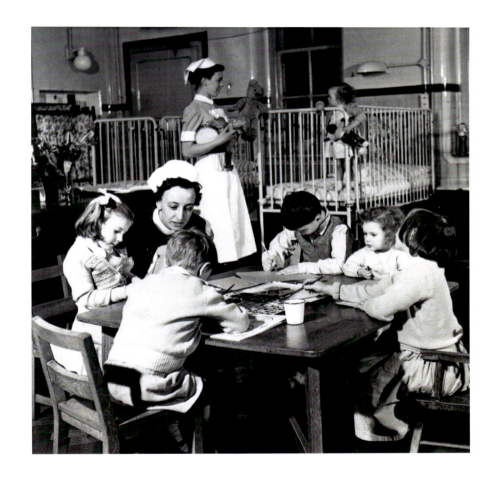
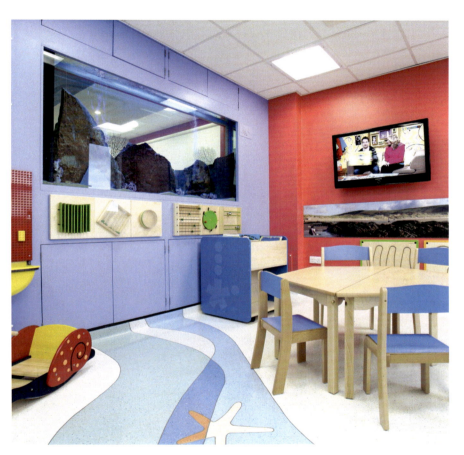

PAEDIATRIC DEPARTMENT

Nurses caring for children in King's paediatric wards in 1959 (left). A contemporary playroom on the Rays of Sunshine Ward in the Variety Children's Hospital (right)

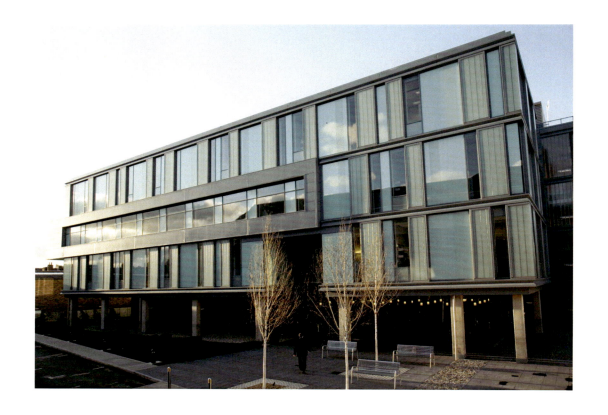

JAMES BLACK BUILDING
Named after the Nobel-winning pharmacologist,
King's College London's £30m research centre
opened in 2007 next to the hospital

MEDICINE THEN
AND NOW

1820s: Brain tumour 'treated' by cupping (suction on the skin, believed to increase blood flow) or counter irritation (mildly inflaming the skin). **Today:** Tumour can be identified by MRI or CT scan and removed in surgery.

1830s: Some patients were hypnotised before operations. Anaesthetic did not exist until ether was first used in 1846. **Today:** General anaesthetic is given by injection or gas.

1840s: Open fractures often resulted in amputation. Surgeon Robert Liston could amputate a limb in 28 seconds. **Today:** Treated with antibiotics and severe fractures can be pinned using a frame (fixator).

1895: X-rays required 25 minutes exposure. **Today:** X-rays take seconds.

1950s: Open-heart surgeons immersed patients in ice-cold water and wrapped them in cooling blankets to induce hypothermia. This increased the time patients could survive without a pumping heart – and could be operated on – to around 15 minutes. **Today:** Heart-lung machines do the work of the heart during surgery. Beating heart surgery immobilises just a small area of the heart for surgery.

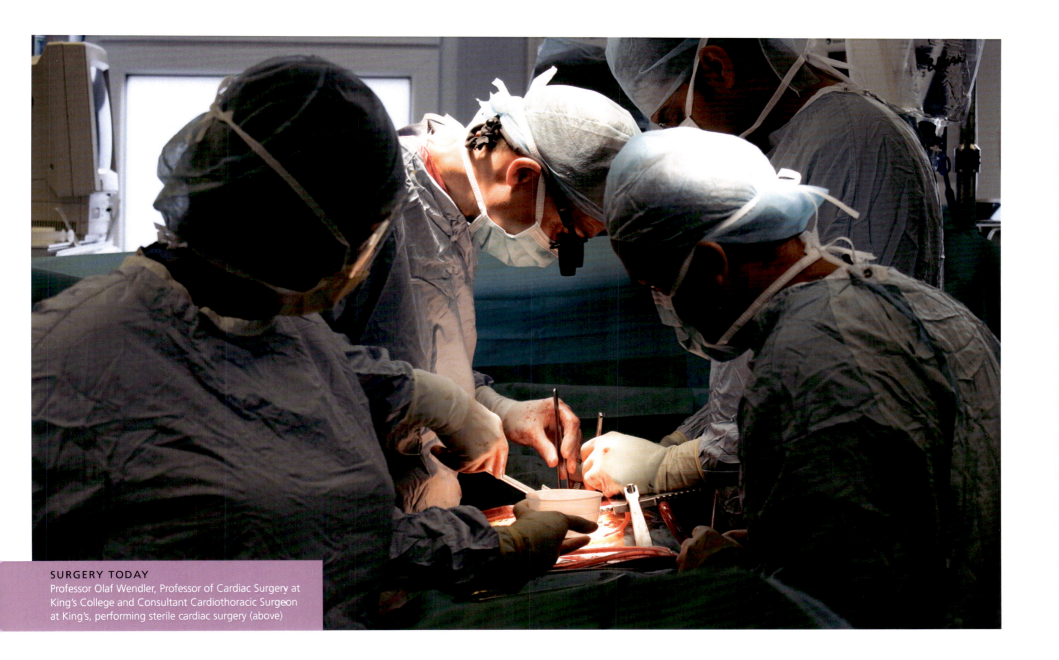

SURGERY TODAY
Professor Olaf Wendler, Professor of Cardiac Surgery at King's College and Consultant Cardiothoracic Surgeon at King's, performing sterile cardiac surgery (above)

KING'S SPECIALITIES UNDER THE MICROSCOPE:
EXPERT PERSPECTIVES

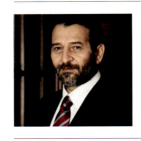

Professor Kypros Nicolaides
Fetal Medicine

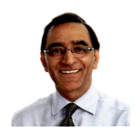

Professor Ghulam Mufti
Haematology

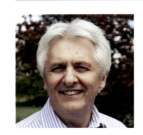

Professor Nigel Heaton
Liver Transplantation

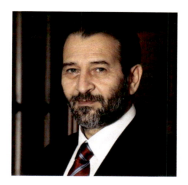

Professor Kypros Nicolaides is King's Professor of Fetal Medicine and the director of the Harris Birthright Research Centre for Fetal Medicine – the first fetal medicine unit in the UK, caring for more than 15,000 patients a year. He is a world-renowned expert in prenatal diagnosis and fetal surgery and director of the Fetal Medicine Centre and Foundation

---

"The Harris Birthright Centre pioneered most of the current methods of fetal surgery: blood transfusions to fetal cells; laser surgery to separate identical twins affected by twin-to-twin transfusion syndrome [TTTS: twins have unequal shares of the placenta and necessary nutrients]; putting balloons in the trachea to treat babies with Congenital Diaphragmatic Hernia [CDH: the diaphragm fails to form correctly, making the abdominal contents push into the baby's chest cavity]. King's also introduced nuchal translucency – a screening technique for Down's Syndrome now used throughout the world.

Recently we've been collaborating on a new method of screening based on cell-free DNA – that's DNA in the maternal blood. This can be used to detect Down's Syndrome and other chromosome abnormalities early and accurately. In the next three to four years I expect all women in England will have this test.

King's is also pioneering imaging methods and molecular biology that will define a person's genetic makeup. Just like Angelina Jolie, the actress who had a double mastectomy because she carries the BRCA1 gene that might kill her in 10 years.

For me, the important thing is how to change prenatal care as practised for the last 90 years. Current care is based on seeing women over the course of their pregnancy and hoping to catch things if they happen. My vision is the opposite; to see women at the beginning of their pregnancy at a supra-specialist centre, to define their risks of different pregnancy complications and define their prenatal care. Preventative principles massively reduce future complications."

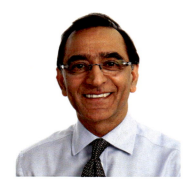

Consultant haematologist **Professor Ghulam Mufti** is Head of Haematological Medicine. When he joined King's 26 years ago, haematology had a handful of inpatient beds and no research. Now it is the leading haematology department in Europe and the UK's largest bone marrow transplant centre, specialising in blood cancers, red blood cell diseases including sickle cell, haemostasis and thrombosis

———

"By common consent, this haematology department is one of the best in Europe. We are a national centre for a number of diseases including bone marrow failure syndromes and myeloid leukaemias. We performed the UK's first bone marrow transplant [in 1986] and through Kingscord pioneered the use of cord blood collection [the blood that remains in the placenta and umbilical cord after a baby is born, which is rich in stem cells].

In the last couple of years we have developed a leukaemia 'vaccine' to reinvigorate the body's immune system; we put specific immune enhancing genes into the leukaemia cells so that the body's immune system recognises the leukaemic cells as foreign and mounts a response against them. We are currently running a clinical trial – a world first.

We are also researching the genetic abnormalities that initiate a leukaemic cell. From the 30,000 genes in the body, we are piecing together the genes that initiate mutations – called 'drivers' – and those that are passengers. That will lead to specific drugs being discovered that kill

off the cells containing driver mutations. This and related biological information identifies the most appropriate therapeutic strategy for leukaemias.

We have a successful leukaemia stem cell research group, which has identified novel therapeutic targets that are currently being progressed into the clinic.

The department is a national/international exemplar for thromboembolic disease and has helped to set national standards for the prevention and treatment of venous thrombosis. The department has a large programme of clinical, translational and basic research in paediatric and adult sickle cell disease, a disease particularly prevalent in south London.

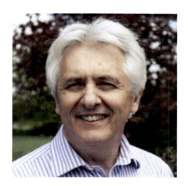

Professor Nigel Heaton is Consultant Liver Transplant Surgeon and Director of Transplant Surgery at King's College Hospital. From a two-bed Liver Failure Unit in 1973 – the first in the world – King's is now the largest liver transplant centre in Europe, with one of the largest children's liver services in the world. It has continually pioneered liver treatment and is breaking new ground with cell transplantation

"In 1965 Roger Williams joined King's. He pioneered liver-based intensive care and transplantation. In 1968, with Sir Roy Calne at Cambridge University, he performed the first liver transplants in the UK. In the early 1970s, King's began its paediatric liver service and that mix of adult and children is very unique in an institution, and very useful for research. In 1993 we became the only centre in the UK to offer living donor transplantation, from parent to child, and then in 1998 from adult to adult. We've now done approaching 200 living donor transplants, making us by far the most active unit in the country.

We began splitting livers – between one child and one adult – in the early 1990s, but now we're trying to split livers for two adults, to develop the full left and right transplantation; for me that remains the final frontier of surgical liver transplantation. King's also has international expertise in auxiliary liver transplantation. We remove half the patient's liver and replace it with a donor-matched half. A year or so downstream we slowly withdraw the immunosuppression drugs [used to prevent the body rejecting the new liver], the transplanted piece of liver shrinks down and disappears and

the patient's own liver grows back. The liver has tremendous regenerative capacity. The advantage is, the patient is not exposed to a lifetime of immunosuppression. That is the key now in terms of longevity post transplantation. We're deciding whether to file a patent for some of the work we're doing around helping livers to regenerate more rapidly. We're the only centre in the country with transplant programmes in both islet cells [for treatment of type 1 diabetes] and hepatocytes [the liver's factory cells]. If we get a young baby with liver failure, instead of replacing their liver we can inject cells through a vein in the tummy button. These cells grow inside the liver and sustain the child to recovery. We can already produce hepatocytes in a soup, which can be injected.

In March 2013 King's began the world's first clinical trials of the OrganOx machine designed by Oxford University. It can keep a liver alive outside the body for up to 24 hours. We can also check how well a liver's working before implanting, and the machine may also be able to resuscitate livers. We think OrganOx will increase the number of livers available for transplantation and that it will be in wider use in around 18 months."

Chapter 7

KING'S COLLEGE HOSPITAL
– ALWAYS A ROYAL HOSPITAL

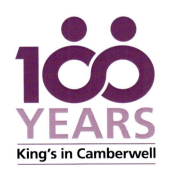

KING'S COLLEGE HOSPITAL
– ALWAYS A ROYAL HOSPITAL

Since King's College was granted a **royal charter by King George IV in 1829,** King's College Hospital has enjoyed close royal links. **Queen Victoria** was the **first patron of the hospital** – then at Lincoln's Inn – and her grandson **George V opened the new hospital at Denmark Hill**. Since then, King's has welcomed many royal visitors

King Edward VII's visit to lay the new hospital's foundation stone in 1909 established a long and distinguished connection with the royal family. On July 26, 1913 King George V and Queen Mary opened the new King's College Hospital at Denmark Hill. Nurses peered down from above the entrance of the new building – now the Hambleden Wing – for a glimpse of the royal couple, and especially Queen Mary's spectacular floral hat. In the 100 years since, King's has enjoyed many royal visits to open new wards, unveil new medical equipment and even to name a cot. In 1929 the Queen Mother – then Duchess of York – visited the children's department and named a cot after her newborn daughter, Princess Elizabeth – now Her Majesty the Queen.

In fact, King's has a strong connection with royal births. Sir William Gilliatt, a King's surgeon who founded the obstetrics and gynaecology department at King's, was obstetrician and gynaecologist to the royal family. The British press door-stepped Sir William before he attended the births of Prince Charles in 1948 and Princess Anne two years later. King's man Sir John Peel then became surgeon-gynaecologist to the Queen and delivered Princes Andrew and Edward. In 1952 on her accession to the throne, the Queen agreed to be Patron of

King's and she made her first visit to the hospital, with Prince Philip Duke of Edinburgh, during her coronation tour in 1953. The Queen returned in 1968 to open the New Ward Block for obstetrics and child health. By this time she had her own young children: Andrew and Edward were just eight and four years old. The *South London Observer* reported how excited patients met the Queen. *"Mrs Edna Horne, 22, from Camberwell, who had just given birth to a baby girl said: 'Her Majesty asked me if I was being well looked after and whether my baby was a boy or girl. It was a great thrill to meet her.'"* And once inside the special intensive care unit, *"the Queen continually asked doctors about how the technical equipment operated."*

Other members of the royal family have made several visits to King's. *British Pathé News* from 1936 shows children and Camberwell locals madly waving flags outside the hospital as the Queen Mother arrived for a tour. She returned in 1958 to open the hospital's new Medical School and saw departments including Medical, Surgical and Chemical Pathology, described somewhat mystically by King's Chairman Lord Normanby in his opening speech as a *"department of modern alchemy, where the search for the philosopher's stone continues."*

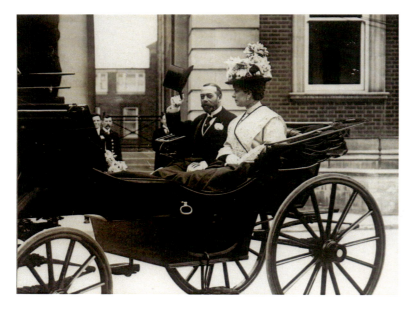

THE ROYAL OPENING
On July 26, 1913 King George V and Queen Mary officially opened the new 300-bed King's College Hospital, greeted by assembled nurses and dignitaries

In 1983 Diana, Princess of Wales opened the Harris Birthright Centre and two years later Anne, the Princess Royal, opened the Variety Children's Hospital.

In 2002, 50 years after becoming patron of King's, the Queen opened the Golden Jubilee Wing. Now in 2013, 100 years after its move to Denmark Hill, King's is looking forward to another royal visit to mark its centenary.

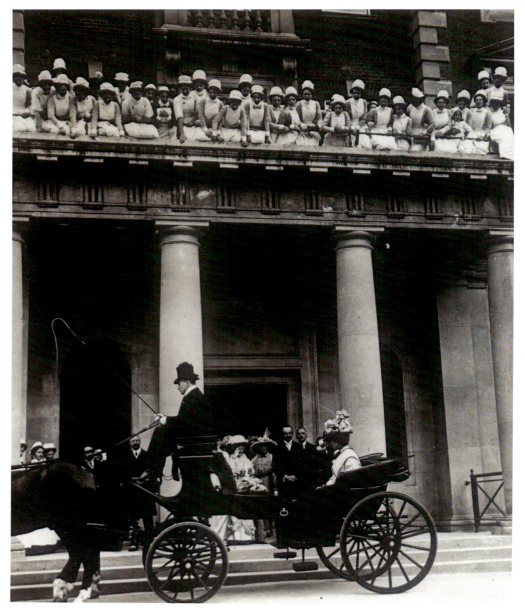

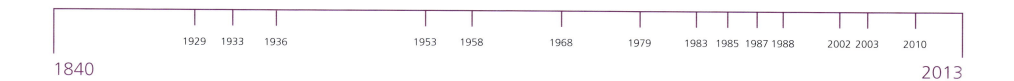
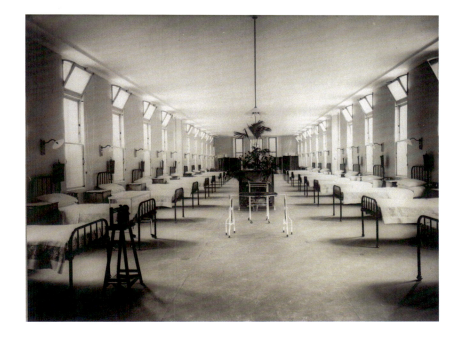

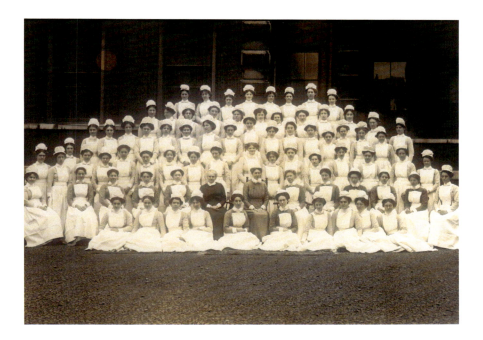

STAFF AT KING'S COLLEGE HOSPITAL
July 1913 – Images of the interior (top left) and official photograph of the King's nursing staff to mark the Royal visit (top right)

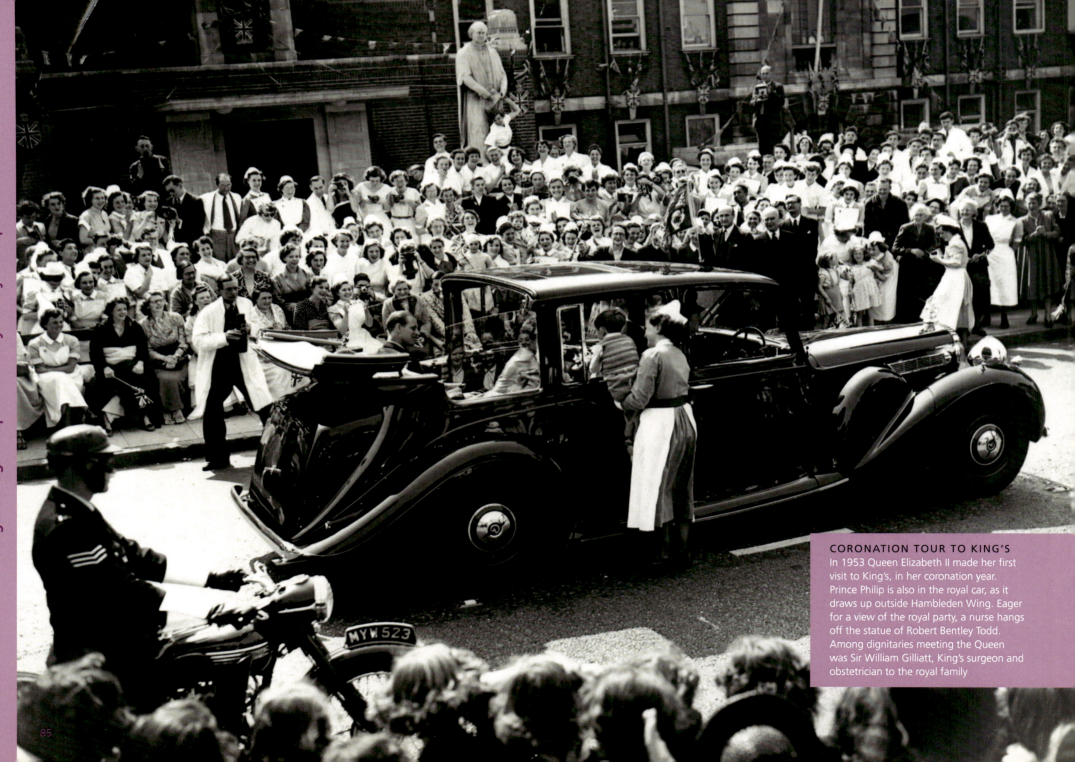

CORONATION TOUR TO KING'S
In 1953 Queen Elizabeth II made her first visit to King's, in her coronation year. Prince Philip is also in the royal car, as it draws up outside Hambleden Wing. Eager for a view of the royal party, a nurse hangs off the statue of Robert Bentley Todd. Among dignitaries meeting the Queen was Sir William Gilliatt, King's surgeon and obstetrician to the royal family

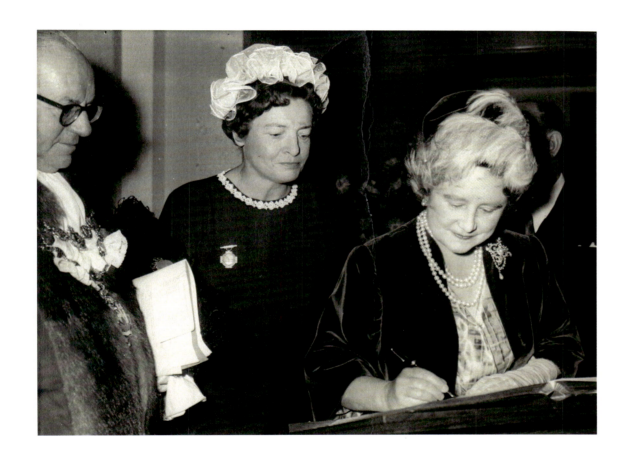

QUEEN MOTHER
The Queen Mother records an official visit
to the hospital in the mid-1950s

KEY ROYAL VISITS

- **1913** On July 26, King George V and Queen Mary officially opened the new 300-bed King's College Hospital

- **1958** Queen Mother opens the Medical School extension

- **1968** The Queen opens the New Ward Block for gynaecology, obstetrics, infertility

- **1979** Queen Mother opens Rayne Institute for research

- **1983** Diana, Princess of Wales opens Harris Birthright Centre

- **1985** Princess Anne opens the Variety Children's Hospital and haematology department

- **1988** Princess Margaret opens the kidney transplant ward

- **2003** Queen Elizabeth II opens the Golden Jubilee Wing

Chapter 8

KING'S IN
THE FUTURE

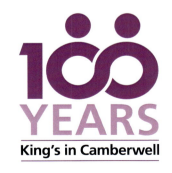

KING'S IN
THE FUTURE

This publication celebrates the achievements of King's and its people over the past 100 years. As an organisation King's has continued to grow to meet the changing needs of its ever-expanding population. In April 2010 King's became one of four Major Trauma Centres in London. And since April 2013 it has led the South East London Kent and Medway Major Trauma Network; 4.5 million people now look to King's for treatment for the most serious and life-threatening injuries

Robert Bentley, Clinical Director, King's Major Trauma Centre, explains the transformation of the A&E department in just three years, including introducing a resident major trauma consultant to receive and review cases 24/7. *"We've aligned the whole hospital along an acute system. King's is no longer a multi-speciality hospital; it's a speciality hospital with teams sharing good practice,"* explains Bentley. *"Everyone signs up to the common vision, 'from roadside to rehab.'*

"We set up pre-alerts so that, in an emergency, the hospital is put on standby to react as quickly as possible to incoming patients," says Bentley. *"We are pioneering patients coming directly to the CT scanner; this aids diagnosis and patients can be simultaneously resuscitated with pre-arranged blood products. This saves time, and time affects outcome."*

The next step for the King's Major Trauma service is a helipad on the roof of Ruskin Wing. Currently, air ambulances land in Ruskin Park and patients are transferred to the resuscitation room in ED by ambulance, which can take a critical extra 20 minutes. And a new Critical Care Unit, with 60 beds, is also in

development, to be built above the existing operating theatre block. *"The extra beds will allow us to honour our responsibility as a major trauma network,"* says Bentley.

"The significance for the local population is that our teams are getting more and more exposure to treating the most severely injured cases. King's has always been bold in adapting to challenges. What we are doing now goes back to our heritage as a major trauma receiving hospital in the First World War."

Despite limited space, expansion at King's continues with the creation of two new 'infill' blocks to house more operating and treatment facilities. This will increase hospital capacity and enable King's to reduce waiting times and provide a better experience for patients and their families.

King's continues to work with its academic partners to create real and lasting benefits for patients and the local community. The new clinical research facility based at the hospital provides a vital modern facility for research teams in

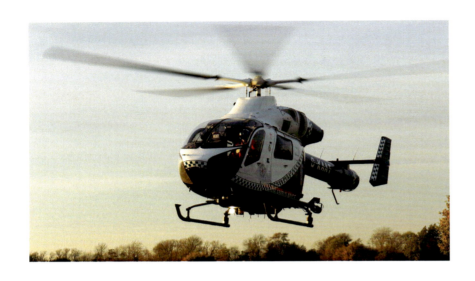

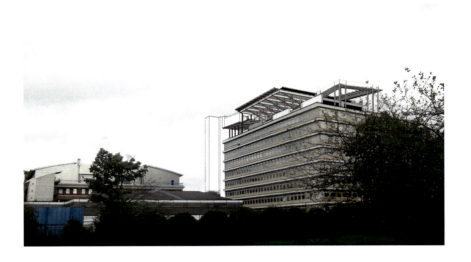

NEW HELIPAD AND CRITICAL CARE UNIT

Air ambulances bringing patients to King's currently land in nearby Ruskin Park (above)
Proposed designs for a new helipad on the roof of the Ruskin Wing (top right) and for the
Critical Care Unit (bottom right)

the area. The facility will focus on stem cell research as well as neurological
and behavioural discrders and enable King's to be at the forefront of new
developments in treatment and care.

King's is proud of its connections with the local community it serves and
takes pride in providing them with the best possible care. As King's looks to
expand its services across south London and surrounding areas, with a focus
on delivering more traditionally hospital-based services in the community, this
is an exciting and innovative time for the hospital. King's looks forward to
building on its successes and continuing to work to provide the best possible
care for patients in the future.

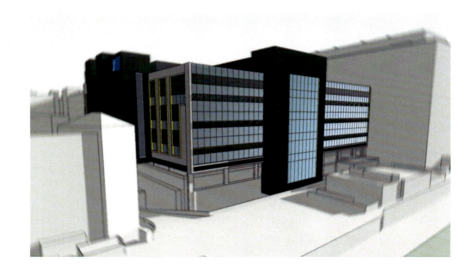

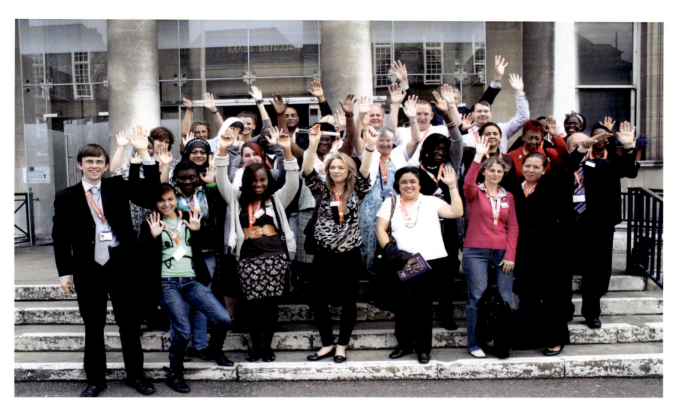

VOLUNTEERS SCHEME
Volunteers celebrate the launch of the scheme in 2012

King's has a special relationship with the people that live in its local community, and this has been demonstrated over the last couple of years with the launch of a new, fundamentally different volunteeriang scheme. The scheme is designed to give local people much needed training and the experience of working within a hospital environment and to give our patients a better experience of their hospital stay by spending time talking to them and helping them find their way around the sometimes complicated systems within the hospital.

King's currently has around 800 volunteers, and has a target of 1,500 across the Hospital. The scheme has been cited by the Government as a positive example of organisations interacting with local communities, and people giving their time to improve the lives of others, and is to be used as a role model for other organisations to follow.

ACKNOWLEDGEMENTS

- King's Collections – King's College London Archives

- Southwark Local History Library

- Lambeth Archive, Minet Library

- Annie Mary Esler interview, p27. Imperial War Museums Collections; © IWM www.iwm.org.uk/collections/item/object/80000555

- Hunterian Museum at the Royal College of Surgeons

- The story of King's College Hospital and its Medical School 1829-1990, editor DJ Britten, 1991

- The Story of King's College Hospital, David Jenkins and Andrew T Stanway, 1968

- The Story of King's College Hospital; TH Whittington talking to Peter Watkins and Geoffrey Davies

- History and development of the Liver Unit – IG McFarlane, ALWF Eddleston, PM Smith,RPH Thompson; Gut Supplement, 1991, BMJ

- Victorian London, The Life of a City 1840-1870, Liza Picard; Phoenix, 2006

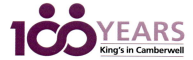

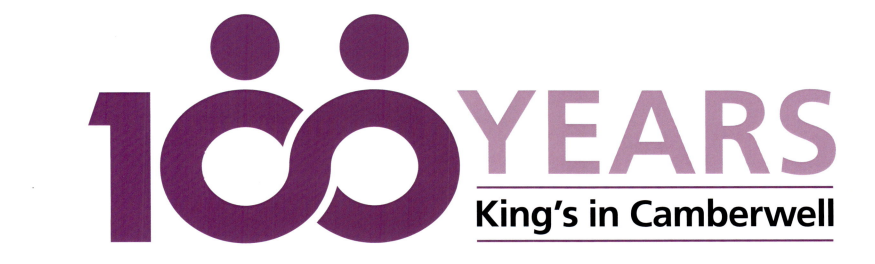